Cure at Home

Dr N. Anantha Raman is a postgraduate (M.D.) in Ayurveda from Bangalore University and has been practising Classical Ayurveda for almost three decades. He has more than 300 articles and successful books like *Mane Oushadhi, Arogya Margadarshi* and *Tonnu Chikitse* to his credit.

Dr A. Karthik is a meritorious medical graduate from the reputed Bangalore Medical College. He has published a number of articles on medical subjects in Kannada and English newspapers. His book on liver disorders has been widely appreciated.

Cure at Home

Dr. N. Anantha Raman
Dr. A. Karthik

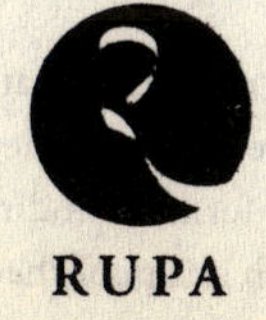

RUPA

Published by
Rupa Publications India Pvt. Ltd 2003
7/16, Ansari Road, Daryaganj
New Delhi 110002

Sales centres:
Allahabad Bengaluru Chennai
Hyderabad Jaipur Kathmandu
Kolkata Mumbai

ISBN: 978-81-716-7655-2

Third impression 2015
10 9 8 7 6 5 4 3

Design: Supriya Saran

Printed at Saurabh Printers, Noida

Contents

Introduction

Man has always been on the look out for medicines to combat diseases. This research has gone through several phases, in his endeavour to find superior remedies. It might have evolved from the discovery of medicinal flora in the local environs, extractions from raw material in the soil and also from animals. In time these discoveries inaugurated various systems of medicine. Our friendly garden and backyard flora together with our very own kitchen provisions gained importance as the impeccable and ever-reliable Home Remedies. This book intends to throw light on some of these simple, effective and time-tested Home Remedies.

Common cold, Much to be told

1

No man on earth till date has escaped common cold. With industrialisation gaining a strong foothold the world over, increasing environmental pollution, stray plants and dust have added fuel to the fire. Common cold usually presents itself with the symptoms of headache, running nose and frequent sneezes.

So, here are our warriors who fight common cold.

TURMERIC

• A piece of turmeric should be held above a flame till it fumes. These fumes are then deeply inhaled, the breath held for a while and then exhaled. The turmeric fumes very effectively combat common cold, open up the blocked nostrils and reduce headache. Also, inhalation of fumes generated by heating a mixture of ragi-powder and turmeric-powder over a flame produces a similar effect. Water should not be consumed for the next two hours as water consumed within this "window-period" magnifies the illness within no time.

• Alternatively, turmeric is ground into a paste which is warmed and applied as a pack over the forehead, in between the eyebrows, along the bridge of the nose and sloping towards both the sides of the nose. This liquefies the thick inspissated mucus that clog the frontal and maxillary sinuses adjoining our nasal passage.

• In addition, powdered turmeric, dissolved in hot milk, and with honey added for taste, makes a very effective beverage. When consumed three times a day, it gets rid of common cold permanently. Since turmeric has excellent immunomodulator and immunity-boosting properties, it makes a perfect medicine for common cold. Addition of honey helps in expulsion of adherent mucus.

TULASI (BASIL)

Sri Tulasi and *Krishna Tulasi* are the two varieties of this plant. Both have indispensable medicinal value. A portion of the plant is cut with stem and leaves. This is crushed and its juice extracted. One teaspoon of this juice mixed with equal quantity of honey is consumed three times a day. *Tulasi* is not only effective against common cold but also prevents a large number of communicable diseases. It is for this reason that this plant made its presence felt in every home in the olden days.

• Alternatively, a handful of *Tulasi* leaves is crushed and placed in a container. Three glasses of water are then boiled and added to the container with the leaves. A lid is placed on the container and left alone till the water cools. Later this water is decanted and consumed three times a day. An oily ingredient of *Tulasi* which resembles camphor in properties is actually responsible for its medicinal value. It is also effective in cases of sore throat because of its soothing effect.

• We all know that clove forms an integral part of traditional medicine. A piece of clove kept in the side of the mouth emanates an oily substance which works wonders in curing cold, headache, sore throat, oral infections and tooth ache. It also prevents further attacks of nasal blocks and common cold.

• In addition, juice extracted from one whole lemon and mixed with equal quantity of warm water should be consumed on an empty stomach. This strengthens immunity and prevents recurrent attacks of common cold.

COUGH

While the same elements causing common cold such as dust, smoke and suspended particles in the air are responsible for a bout of cough, consumption of polluted water is an important cause. Sore throat, change in the voice and throat irritation are the common companions of cough. Cough could be dry or productive (that which brings forth sputum or phlegm). Since the sound produced by cough resembles that produced by a bronze vessel, cough is termed *Kaasa* in Sanskrit.

The remedies for cough are as follows:

• Catechu is powdered and half a teaspoon of the same is thoroughly stirred and dissolved in warm water. The resulting solution is taken orally to fill the whole of the mouth cavity (Do not drink). The chin is then elevated so that the face turns upwards. After two minutes of holding the solution in the mouth in that position, it is spat out. This procedure is repeated thrice daily to ward off sore throat, cold, headache and irritant cough. Catechu possesses astringent and hygroscopic properties which cause expectoration of the thick and inspissated mucus in the throat and mouth-cavity.

• The roots of liquorice are cut into small pieces. When kept in the sides of the mouth they release their juice that relieves throat irritation and sore throat. This keeps cough under control.

In addition, half a teaspoon of liquorice powder consumed with honey keeps cough in control. In cases of dry cough, this powder is mixed with half a cup of water and consumed to get promising results.

• The juice extracted from a combination of black pepper and some crystal salt placed in the mouth takes care of productive cough. The "hot-n-spicy" character of these spices relieve throat discomfort caused by cough.

• Ten raisins are allowed to soak in half a cup of hot water for a while. Then, they are squeezed to release their ingredients and the resulting solution is consumed three times a day to get rid of cough and associated weakness.

• Ruta leaves, *tulasi* leaves and thick leaved lavender leaves are taken in equal quantities. The combination is placed in a betel leaf which is folded and roasted in a pan. When completely dry, it is thoroughly crushed and water added to extract its juice. The juice is then consumed with equal quantity of honey thrice daily to obtain express relief from nagging cough.

The simple home-remedies stated above are of help to both adults and children alike, but children (upto 12 years) should consume half the dose given to adults. A weaker immune system renders children more susceptible to these illnesses than adults. Hence, some over-enthusiastic parents tend to keep their children wrapped up in woollens throughout the year. This is a great deterrent to the development of a strong immune system and also renders them highly sensitive to diseases due to trivial weather and seasonal variations. Hence, children should always wear light cotton clothes and must resort to woollens only during the winter season.

Following are the precautionary measures to be used in the case of children.

• One teaspoon of eucalyptus oil added to a mugful of hot water is poured on the infant's body after his bath. The essence of this oil leaves a lasting effect on the tender skin of the infant and this acts as an impermeable barrier to the common cold viruses. Eucalyptus oil is also used in steam inhalations for common cold and nasal blocks. It is an indispensable ingredient of several pain-relief balms commercially available.

• Garlic is crushed and a few drops of its juice extracted. Two drops of this juice mixed with equal quantity of honey makes a perfect remedy for severe illnesses in children.

• The sweet flag root, widely used in child health care, is burnt over a flame. The burnt root is then ground in water to obtain a paste. Quarter teaspoon of this paste is mixed with a little honey and fed to the child early in the morning. This medicine not only cures cold but also increases digestive power.

• The importance of honey as a medicine has long remained unquestioned. According to Ayurveda, "Honey is nectar for your little sunny." Regular intake of honey by growing children provides much needed nutrition. In addition it has anti-cold and immunity-boosting properties.

Ageing is a march towards a second childhood in the sense that the strength of the immune system diminishes with age. Hence, the incidence of cough and cold increases. In addition to the above remedies, the elderly must stay away from venturing out in cold weather and also avoid crowded, dusty and polluted surroundings. Dry gooseberry when powdered and consumed at the rate of one teaspoon in a cup of warm water, thrice daily, wards off weakness and prevents recurrent attacks of cold.

All the home remedies suggested above are effective for all age groups. But, if in case, the common cold does not resolve within three days, the guidance of a qualified doctor is essential.

NAGGING COLD AND NOSE BLOCKS

An attack of cold and nose block that is undeterred by any of the above may probably be due to a structural defect or an additional growth of tissue in the nose. This may be due to a deviation in the bridge (septum) of the nose or a polyp. Hence, the help of an ENT surgeon is advisable and a surgery too, if need be.

Some precautionary measures are:

- Wearing masks in polluted environs.

- Clean the nostrils in warm water four times a day.

- Steam inhalation with deep breathing and exhaling from the mouth.

- Application of a pack of warmed turmeric-paste in between the eyebrows.

In addition, the following home remedies come in handy:

- Turmeric is powdered well and half a teaspoon of the powder is dissolved in half a cup of hot water with some sugar to taste. This is consumed thrice daily. Turmeric has antiseptic and anti-cold properties.

• *Tulasi* leaves are crushed thoroughly and their juice is extracted. One teaspoon of this juice with equal quantity of honey consumed three times a day keeps cough and common cold at bay.

• A lemon is squeezed and the juice thus obtained is mixed with equal quantity of hot water and consumed early in the morning on an empty stomach. This boosts appetite and immunity as well.

These remedies work wonders when the patient practises deep breathing exercises (Prãnãyãma) regularly for at least a month.

Why does ear discharge accompany long-standing cold?

A long-standing cold provides enough time for invading micro-organisms to gain a strong foothold. These invariably spread, leading to infections of the eye and the ear. Hence prevention of common cold is of prime importance.

The suggested remedies for these conditions are:
• Indian sarasaparila roots are ground into a very fine powder. Half a teaspoon of this powder mixed in a cup of hot water is consumed three times a day. This herb has an anti-microbial action and cures cold and ear discharge.

• Two black pepper seeds are powdered and taken with half a teaspoon of turmeric powder and two *tulasi* leaves. The whole mixture is added to a container holding half a cup each of milk and water. The solution is brought to boil over a flame till all the water content vapourises. The resulting solution is decanted, a spoon of honey is added, and consumed three times a day.

• Warm water is held in the mouth and the chin is elevated with the face facing upwards. After holding for a while, the water is spat out. This cleanses the tube connecting the ear and the throat (eustachian tube) and hence controls ear infections.

But, all said and done, the advice of an ENT specialist is always indispensable, if the problems persist.

2

Diseases of the Skin

The human body is an incredible creation made of bones, muscles, nerves and blood vessels. The bones occupy the innermost compartment and are held together by tendons, ligaments and muscles. Blood vessels make way in between, along and among these structures. The skin acts as a protective covering for all these structural organs. In addition to security vigilance, the skin also strikes the right balance in maintaining body-water and regulating body-temperature. Our skin has two layers with sweat glands, sebum (oil) secreting sebaceous glands and hair follicles interspersed between. Excess body salts are excreted in the sweat thereby maintaining electrolyte balance. The sweat from the skin vapourises on the skin surface which has a cooling effect. Hence, by varying the amount of sweat excretion depending on climate, the skin maintains the body-temperature at a constant level of 37°C (98.6°F) irrespective of external temperature. Our brain controls all these functions. The sense of touch, pain, heat, cold, vibration etc., are all felt when these stimuli are carried as impulses by the nerves in the skin to the brain. The brain being the highest seat of consciousness, responds to these stimuli after which we feel and understand the kind of sensation.

Though the skin performs the same functions in all human beings, it projects diversity when it comes to complexion. The complexion of an individual is largely determined by climate, type of food consumed and hereditary influences. The pigment "Melanin" gives colour to the skin. Greater its content, darker the individual and the lesser its presence, fairer the individual.

Consumption of nutritious food and regular baths are the keys to a glowing healthy skin. There are several factors leading to skin diseases that spoil its natural beauty. Hence, Ayurveda describes all skin diseases under a common generic term *Kushta. Krishnathi Vapuhu Ithi Kushtaha*—this means that the term *Kushta* was coined for those diseases that alter the skin colour, giving it an ugly appearance. Though the term *Kushta* scientifically refers to the debilitating disease leprosy, in Ayurveda it refers to all skin diseases leading to a darker skin.

The cause of all these conditions are varied and many, as stated below:

• Prolonged intake of food having completely opposite properties (such as too hot and extremely cold) is a major deterrent to skin health. A cup of cold curd at the end of a heavy (hot) meal would show up as skin problems. Withholding nature's call for too long increases toxic substances in the blood that forms a thriving ground for micro-organisms causing skin diseases. Hence, imbalance in our biological clock is the root cause.

A large chunk of skin diseases are caused by bacteria, fungi and allergens. Some of them like psoriasis, vitiligo, ringworm and the like are curable only under a dermatologist's supervision.

The effective home remedies for some common skin problems are as follows:

SHEETHAPITTHA: URTICARIA (ALLERGIC CONDITION)

Urticaria is described as *Sheethapittha* in Ayurveda. In some hypersensitive (allergy prone) individuals, the contact of skin with snow, rainwater, dew or a cool breeze results in intense itching . In addition, certain kinds of food especially eggs, wheat, meat, corn, certain cereals etc., detergents and soaps may also trigger violent itching. An individual may be allergic to different kinds of substances depending on his/her own hereditary character and body constitution. It is widely known that allergic tendencies run in families. Hence, a scientist has stated thus, "Every life under the sun is sensitive to some substance including sunlight!!"

Urticaria is characterised by violent red rashes on the skin and itching, followed by a terrible burning sensation. It may also be associated with other allergic manifestations like difficulty in breathing, chest pain, gastroenteritis, eye irritation etc. Urticaria in children is also suggestive of a heavy worm infestation.

The following home remedies are useful:

• Sandal paste is applied over the affected area of the skin and left for a while. Later it is washed away in lukewarm water. Similarly, white clay can also be used.

• Thick leaved lavender is an edible green leafy vegetable widely available. Some leaves are taken, crushed thoroughly and the juice is extracted. The juice is applied over the areas of skin affected and left for a while after which it is washed away.

• A handful of cumin seeds is roasted over a frying-pan with a pinch of pure ghee added to it. After a few minutes, equal quantity of jaggery is added to make a perfect medicine that immediately controls itching on consumption.

• The roots of liquorice are powdered thoroughly. Half a teaspoon of this powder mixed with quarter teaspoon of turmeric powder is dissolved in half a cup of hot milk and consumed three times a day. This brings down urticaria and its accompanying itching and burning sensations.

ECZEMA

This skin disorder is termed *Gajakarna* in Ayurveda which translates into "Elephant ear" in English. The reason behind coining this term is that it is a troublesome itch concentrated in a part of the body which later turns very dark and thick resembling the texture of an elephant's ear.

This disorder is commonly seen around joints, soles, foot, areas of the body where the skin folds like upper thigh, elbow, knee etc. Eczema may be present either in a dry form or an exudative form. The disorder makes frequent appearances during rainfall and winter. The disease is also exacerbated by consumption of food that have properties opposed to the season. The person has to make a herculean effort to resist the violent itching associated with the disorder. The patient is advised to wash the affected part with soap and water three to four times a day and keep it dry and clean.

The home remedies that are helpful in this disorder are:

- A lime is crushed and the juice extracted. A turmeric piece is ground well in this juice to obtain a paste. This paste when applied to the affected parts three to four times a day gives remarkable results due to the anti-allergic and antiseptic properties of turmeric. Inspite of the burning sensation, this treatment helps in the peeling off of the affected skin and facilitates growth of healthy new skin.

- Coconut shell is burnt till it is charred. The charred shell is powdered and mixed with sufficient coconut oil to make a paste. When this paste is applied to the affected parts, it relieves the intense itching.

- Radish seeds are powdered well and a teaspoon is mixed with a little quantity of sour curds. The resulting mixture is allowed to stand overnight. The next morning, this paste is applied to the affected body parts, left for a while and later washed away. Not only does this relieve the itching, but also helps in the thinning of the tough skin that finally peels off.

• Catechu is powdered well and a quarter teaspoon of this powder mixed with equal quantity of honey is consumed three times a day. This helps in reducing itching and also in blood purification.

• Two handfuls of neem leaves are crushed well to extract the juice. Half a teaspoon of this juice is added to half a cup of water. The resulting solution is heated over a flame till it vapourises and the volume is reduced to half. This solution is consumed along with some honey on an empty stomach.

WHITE PATCHES AND CHILBLAINS

The large white patches that appear on the face, back, shoulder and chest are termed as chilblains. These may sometimes itch.

The home remedies that come in handy are:

• The root of sweet flag plant is powdered well. One teaspoon of this powder is mixed with a little butter milk to make a paste. This is applied overnight. It is then washed away in lukewarm water the following day.

• The juice extracted from crushed lime is applied to the chilblains and left for a while. A little later it is washed away. Similarly, the dried skin of a lime fruit is powdered, mixed with equal amount of round zedoary and double its quantity of besan flour. This mixture is rubbed over the chilblain affected skin and washed away after a while. This makes a perfect mix of medicine that cures chilblains.

• Indian sarasaparilla root is powdered well. One teaspoon of this powder is added to half a cup of water to make a solution which when consumed thrice daily, cures chilblains.

CORNS

It is a very painful condition affecting the toes and soles, particularly those of the overweight. It is usually present as hard nodular growth of the skin.

Many people in their frustration voluntarily try to cut it off using unsterilised shaving blades. This can in turn cause them more harm than good, leading to septic infection. Some simple tips go a long way in helping such patients.

• The affected leg/s is/are dipped in a bucket of hot water for a few minutes at night. It is later wiped dry and gingiley oil is massaged gently over the corn. This relieves the pain and softens the layer of skin.

• The juice extracted from onion when applied to the corn, twice daily, takes care of pain.

• Plumbago roots are ground well in lime juice extract and the paste obtained is applied over the corn. This softens the skin making the corn fall off.

WARTS

Warts are small external growths of the skin, dark in colour mainly affecting the face and the neck. This is commonly seen among the obese. Though warts do not cause any sort of burning or itching whatsoever, they cause great concern to the beauty conscious. They can find solace in the following home remedies:

• A potato is cooked well in water. When cooking is complete, the water left over is applied to the warts. This makes a great medicine.

• As in the case of corns, plumbago roots are ground well in lime juice extract and the paste thus obtained is applied to the warts.

• In folk-medicine, a strand of hair obtained from a horse's tail is tied tightly along the root of the wart. Amazingly, the warts wither away in a few days. The scientific reason behind the success of this treatment is that, a hair tied tightly around the root of a wart cuts off its blood supply leading to its fall.

But a horse's tail is not easily available. An alternative home remedy based on the same principle is as follows:

• A piece of fine thread is soaked in lime juice

extract and a little turmeric powder is smeared along its length. This thread when tied to the root of the wart makes it fall off in a few days without leaving any scars.

HOW TO GET RID OF DARK PATCHES?

Facial patches dark in colour called "melasma" never itch or pain or cause any sort of illness. They may remain for months together and may fade out very slowly.

But a mirror says it all and hence it is a matter of concern for many.

The home remedies that help are:

- A mixture of round zedoary, sandal paste and green gram flour is used for bathing instead of soap.

- Prolonged exposure to sunlight is avoided as it increases the darkness of the affected skin. Hence, a cap or an umbrella should be used.

- One whole chebulic myloboron is boiled well in a cup of milk and dried. This dried nut is again boiled in milk and the procedure is repeated five times in a row. This is finally dried and ground well in water to make a paste. This paste is applied to the darkened areas of skin for a minimum period of two months to produce results.

The colour of our skin is determined by heredity,

our lifestyle and the climatic conditions we live in. Foreigners commonly take sunbath on the sea shores which tans the skin. But, all said and done, no food or medicine can ever change the natural colour of our skin.

3

Joint Pain

Joint pain is a term that sends a chill down many a spine. Hence, it is extremely important to check our posture while standing, sitting or lying down, failing which we are bound to go down with joint pain. If this joint pain remains neglected, it can cripple the body for a lifetime. Though this condition is common in old age, it can strike at any age. The bones lend support and give a definite shape to our body. Several bones join together in a specific pattern to form the skeleton. Movements occur at the points where two bones meet called the joint. The joints are protected by a thick capsule which holds the bones together. The opposing bony surfaces at the joint are covered by a layer of spongy substance called cartilage. There is a joint space between the opposing bones which is filled by a lubricating substance called synovial fluid that prevents friction between bones during joint movement.

There are several types of joints in our body depending on the type of movements carried out. The various causes of joint pain are listed below:

• Over-exertion at any joint leads to extreme wear and tear of the lubricating substances and the cartilage and makes the joint extremely painful and immobile.

• Certain professions like those of traffic policemen, bus conductors etc. demand long hours of standing in an erect posture. The joint yields to intense stress leading to pain in the knee and the calf.

• Infections may spread to the joint from the surrounding areas and cause sickening joint-pain.

• Direct trauma to the joint may lead to a tear in the capsule and cartilage leading to intense pain.

• Sedentary lifestyle, either induced by lethargy or a chronic illness is deleterious to joint health and invariably ends in painful joints.

PAIN IN THE NECK

Neck pain invariably affects some professionals like journalists, bank employees, computer professionals, accountants, clerks and the like, who work long hours with the neck bent down. In addition, the pain even travels down to affect the shoulder and upper arm.

Neck exercises and protection of neck from exposure to the cold are invaluable in controlling neck pain.

The home remedies that provide relief are:

- Sufficient quantity of gingiley oil is massaged gently round the neck. A little later, a handful of whole black gram is taken and dry-heated in a frying pan over a strong flame. These heated seeds are bound in a clean piece of cloth and hot fomentation is applied to the massaged area.

- The leaves of ruta plant are thoroughly cleaned under running water and crushed well. A handful of these crushed leaves are added to a pan holding a cup measure of gingiley oil and the mixture is fried over a low flame. This is well decanted. The oil thus obtained is massaged from the neck down the shoulder to the upper arm. This increases the local blood circulation and relieves pain.

- A piece of ginger, a whole garlic and Kulinjan (Rashme) are crushed together. Three cups of water are added and the mixture is brought to boil over a low flame. With vapourisation, the solution is reduced to half of its previous volume and decanted. Half a cup of this solution consumed three times a day relieves the muscle-spasm and cures neck pain.

- A freshly cut piece of stem of the tinospora creeper and an equal quantity of ginger are crushed together to extract the juice. One teaspoon of this juice consumed three times a day relieves long standing neck pain.

BACK PAIN / ACHE

Back pain invariably affects a majority of the middle-aged and elderly population.

Prolonged assumption of faulty postures, lack of exercise and obesity are the prime causes of backache. If people working long hours seated, do not assume an erect posture, they can be sure of excruciating backache due to the concentration of the whole body weight on the lower spine. This in turn lays great stress on the nerves of the spinal cord causing additional pain in the legs. Also, the lack of exercise weakens the muscle of the back causing backache. In case of obesity, those extra pounds of fat decorating the expanding waistline, press upon the spinal nerves, causing pain.

In addition, back pain is also experienced by people who are very anaemic (pale) and also by women during their monthly menstrual periods.

The most effective and time-tested home remedies for back pain are:

- Wheat grains are slowly pre-heated over a low flame in an iron pan. These grains are then powdered and one teaspoon of this powder is consumed two times a day with honey, making a perfect medicine for backache and lethargy.

• A spoon of dill (Sabbasige) seeds are powdered well and to this are added two spoons of gingiley oil. This mixture is ground well to obtain a paste which when applied and massaged locally relieves backache.

• A whole garlic (with its outer skin peeled off) is crushed and ground well. To this is added an equal quantity of cumin seeds, ginger and powdered pepper. Long pepper & rock salt are also powdered and added to the above mixture in equal quantities. A small quantity of asafoetida is heated over a pan, powdered and added to the mixture. All the above ingredients are thoroughly mixed to a dough-like consistency. It is then made into pills, about the size of pepper. One pill each in the morning and night consumed with a cup of hot water drives away even the toughest of backaches.

KNEE PAIN

Our knees bear the brunt of the whole body weight when we assume an erect posture. A pain in the knee can be due to several reasons. Prime among these is being overweight and leading a sedentary lifestyle.

In addition, an infection in the knee joint may cause septic arthritis.

An auto-immune (destructive to self) disease process in the knee leads to rheumatoid arthritis. This is termed *Amavata* in Ayurveda.

When the knee joint is over-used, as in case of manual labourers, athletes etc., it leads to wear and tear. A similar process occurs in the elderly, leading to a change in the structural architecture of joints and friction between opposing bony surfaces during movement. This goes by the name of osteoarthritis, referred to as *Sandhi Vata* in Ayurveda.

The pain in the knee due to any of the above causes responds remarkably to the following home remedies, but only in the initial stages. Long standing pain always needs expert care:

• A handful of mustard seeds are ground well in water and later heated over a good flame. The medicine thus prepared is applied to the knee joint twice daily. This increases the blood flow in and around the joint, thereby bringing down pain and swelling. Likewise, the medicine made by crushing sesbania leaves or drum stick leaves, when applied to the knee, provides similar results.

• Application of local heat is indispensable in the treatment of any type of pain. A requisite amount of clean sand is heated over a high flame in an iron pan. This is then tied in a piece of cloth and local heat is applied over and around the knee.

• Calatropis leaves are cleaned under running water and adequate quantity of mustard oil is smeared over them. The leaves are then heated in a pan, and applied over the knee, thus providing local heat. This wards off both pain and swelling.

• Kulinjan, ginger, black cumin seeds are taken in equal quantities and powdered well. To one spoon of this powder are added three cups of water and the mixture is brought to boil over a low flame. When the solution vapourises and is reduced to half its original volume, it is decanted and consumed three times a day.

• Three spoons of ghee, two spoons of castor oil and one spoon of gingiley oil are mixed and brought to boil over a pan. This mixture when massaged around the knee alleviates the pain. This has proven efficacy, especially in the case of osteoarthritis.

DRAGGING PAIN IN THE LEGS

Certain people experience an excruciating pain radiating from the lower back, down the thigh right upto the corresponding foot. This pain is termed as "sciatica". This is due to the irritation and pressure effect upon the sciatic nerve which travels from the spinal cord in the lower back, down the thigh, branching right upto the foot. This is termed *Gridhrasivā.*

Gridhra means vulture in Sanskrit. A keen observation of a vulture walking on the ground reveals that the bird involuntarily drags one of its legs held straight, across the ground.

A patient suffering from "sciatica" also keeps the

affected leg straight and draws it across the ground while walking. Isn't it an excellent simile? This disorder can be set right by the assumption of erect posture while standing and sitting and by controlled exercise.

• A piece of dry bark of the drumstick tree is crushed well and to a spoon of this is added quarter spoon of cumin seeds. In addition three cups of water are added and the mixture is brought to boil till it vapourises to half its volume. The solution is decanted and a pinch of asafoetida and rocksalt are added to it and consumed three times a day.

• Coconut pulp is scraped out and squeezed well to extract its milk. To this is added an equal quantity of lime juice extract and the mixture is gently massaged over the affected joint parts. The coconut extract replenishes the nerve energy and the lime-extract improves local blood circulation. This causes dramatic reversal of symptoms.

• The leaves of the *Dhatura* plant (a stray plant) are washed well, crushed and the juice is extracted. The juice is gently massaged over the affected areas.

An increase in the stretch forces in the outer part of the elbow due to frequent outward swing, like actions of the hand and upper arm in tennis players, leads to a condition called tennis elbow. This may also manifest itself in those who write voraciously. Care should be taken not to lift heavy weights or to sleep with the arm under the head, as these can only make matters worse.

The most effective home remedies for tennis elbow are:

1. A pinch of powdered camphor is added to a small quantity of eucalyptus oil which is gently massaged over the elbow. And the very next moment, the pain is gone!

2. Basil leaves and pepper are mixed and ground in equal quantities. Quarter spoon of this mixture, with a little ghee added, is consumed twice dsaily to obtain lasting relief.

The lean and the obese

4

Well built implies being well fed and it means being well off too! This notion seems to have made a deep impact on the minds of many, especially parents. These days, parents are a worried lot. They are at their wits end trying to figure out the best nutrition regime for their children. Their children either eat too less or too much and striking a perfect balance is a herculean task indeed. In many cases it is the former complaint that rules. In addition, peer pressure, cut–throat competition and obvious comparisons between friends have very serious effect on the child's psychosocial and physical health.

The physical appearance of a person is to a large extent determined by heredity, lifestyle, food intake and physical exertion. A handful of cases might be due to hormonal disturbances, diseases of the digestive system, psychological disorders and the like.

In recent years, over-cautious parents, desirous of seeing their children plump and well built, seek medical advice at the drop of a hat. They usually ask for prescriptions for some health tonic that might add a few kilos and make their child look healthy. It is for this reason that pharmacies are flooded with attractive nutritional supplements and the multinationals are laughing all the way to the bank. This is in fact a bane for children who are otherwise perfectly healthy, but are lean due to their genetic make-up.

A march against nature always ends in disaster. Hence, an otherwise perfectly healthy but lean person does not need a health tonic. A saying in Ayurveda states: *Karshyameva Varam Sthoulyath* which means "It is a boon to be lean rather than obese", because, the obese are more prone to disease than the lean.

GUIDELINES ON PUTTING ON WEIGHT

According to Ayurveda, only an individual who has lost weight due to physical or psychological diseases and increased physical exertion as in the case of manual labourers, farmers, athletes and the like, is eligible to consume medicines that increase body weight. The same is indicated for pregnant women, post-partum women, young children and the elderly, only in case they are anaemic (pale). Due to increased expenditure of energy during summer months, these formulations are indicated for normal healthy people in summer only.

Ayurveda advises the following regimen for those

who desire to gain weight:

• Consumption of plenty of milk and meat (if non-vegetarian).

• Foods rich in ghee and oil.

• Sweets in the daily diet.

• Frequent oil baths.

• Increased hours of sleep.

All these activities make one gain weight. The following home remedies bring added results:

• Fresh, frothing buffalo milk when applied and gently massaged over the face, not only gives a glowing complexion but also prevents sunken cheeks. It nourishes the facial muscles and helps them grow.

• A cup of wheat flour is mixed with an equal quantity of powdered bark of bastard teak tree. To this are added requisite quantities of water, ghee and finely powdered sugar. The whole mixture is heated over a low flame and a thick paste is made. One spoon of this paste followed by a cup of hot milk, consumed twice daily, increases body weight.

• It is well-known that black gram has all properties of meat. Whole black gram is warmed over a low flame and powdered. One spoon of this powder is added to a cup of milk. Raisins with sugar are added to it. The mixture is heated to a thick consistency. When this is consumed twice daily, the body adds weight.

Though ash gourd is a vegetable rich in water-content, it also has weight increasing properties. This vegetable is peeled and grated. The final product is squeezed out of its water content and dry heated in a pan with a little ghee added. An equal quantity of sugar is added to this and a paste is prepared. After the paste cools down, an equal quantity of sugar is added again and mixed well into the paste. One spoon of this jam followed by a cup of hot milk is consumed twice daily to add on body weight. Asparagus roots or withania roots, when used in place of ash gourd, have a similar effect on the body.

OBESITY

The above mentioned disorder is just one face of the coin. The other face is truly nightmarish as it has a deleterious effect on one's health. The fact remains that obesity is the root cause of some of the worst ailments of man like diabetes, heart disease, arteriosclerosis (narrowing of blood vessels) etc.

Statistical evidence show that women are more prone to obesity than men. Psychological disorders ending in alcoholism is an indisputable cause of obesity in men. Unscrupulous consumption of high calorie food and hereditary factors also determine obesity. A weight that is ten percent over and above that corresponding to one's age and height is the prime indication to start losing weight.

A balanced diet and an exercise regimen to suit one's age is a perfect recipe for a trim figure. In fact, weight loss is prescribed not only for healthy obese individuals but also for patients with chronic diseases like diabetes, psoriasis etc.

As experience suggests, one's appetite increases in winter. Lack of exercise and a full stomach adds several kilos and a visible paunch. Hence, indoor exercises are recommended in winter.

The following measures are suggested in Ayurveda to reduce weight:

• The part of the body with excess fat deposition is rinsed in lukewarm water several times in a day. This melts down that extra fat.

• A meal is skipped twice anytime during a week and hot water is consumed frequently.

• Exercise suitable for age and sex is a must for all age groups. One should exercise till he/she sweats adequately. Exposure to the early rays of the sun and practising deep breathing exercises in open lush green environment help in weight reduction. Consumption of horse gram, jowar, corn, green gram, the water floating on curds allowed to stand for long, and honey in the routine diet helps one shed a few kilos.

In addition, the following home remedies give the final touches to a shapely figure:

• The seeds of chebulic myloboron, beleric

myloboron and gooseberry are extracted and powdered well. This powder mixture is mixed with a little water to make a paste which is applied to those parts of the body with excess fat deposition. After a while a warm water bath is taken. This melts down excess fat deposits.

• The stem of tinospora creeper is crushed to extract the juice. Three spoons of this juice is mixed with equal quantity of pure honey and consumed early in the morning on an empty stomach.

• A herb called nut grass grows abundantly in agricultural fields. This herb is washed thoroughly in running water and adequately dried in sunlight. It is then powdered well. The processed form of this herb is also available at the local Pansari-shop. One teaspoon of the above powder is dissolved in a cup of hot water and consumed thrice daily after food. In addition to reducing obesity, it also relieves the joint pain associated with excessive weight.

• The seeds of emblic myloboron plant are powdered well and filtered over a clean piece of cloth to obtain a very fine powder. One spoon of fine powder mixed with honey is consumed three times a day to get beneficial results.

• Chebulic myloboron nut is crushed to remove the seed and is later powdered. To this is added an equal quantity of old jaggery. One spoon of the mixture dissolved in a cup of hot water is consumed three times a day. In addition to shedding excess fat, this also reduces breathlessness and constipation that are the common complaints of obese people. Finally, there are no alternatives to a strict diet and regular exercise in order to sculpt an enviable figure.

5 Home remedies for children

Today's children are tomorrow's citizens. Hence, the health of children in the long run determines a nation's health. There is a media hype trying to make the public aware of the need for efficient child care. In addition, vaccinations, modern diagnostic procedures and instruments, special paediatric medicines and surgical techniques have strengthened paediatric care. Ayurveda had laid stress on child health as early as two thousand years ago. *Kaumara bhrithya* dealing with paediatrics is one of the eight major branches in Ayurveda. The great sage Kashyapa has described in his masterpiece (text) *Kashyapa Samhitha*, the preventive health care of children from infancy to maturity, the various diseases affecting them and cures for the same. As a child feeds mainly on milk from infancy to one year of age, this period was suitably termed as *Ksheerada* (*Ksheera* in Sanskrit means milk). Likewise, a child feeds on milk, semi–solid and certain solid food from one to four years of age and hence this period was termed *Ksheerannada* (Ksheera+Anna = Milk + Cooked rice). As described in Ayurveda, the mode of treatment differs in each of the above age groups.

Mother's milk contains several immunity-boosting factors and nutritive proteins that are easily digestible by the neonate. On the contrary, cow's milk has proteins which the infant cannot digest and hence causes milk-intolerance. Hence, mother's milk is compulsory for the first one year. If in case the mother fails to produce enough milk, saunf leaves and bottle gourd must be added to her diet. Also, asparagus roots should be powdered well, one spoon of the powder dissolved in a cup of hot milk and consumed three times a day.

In addition, the time tested home remedies for specific diseases in children are as follows:

MILK INTOLERANCE

- One whole elaichi is pricked with a sterilised needle and held against a flame till it is burnt. When charred it is converted into powder. The infant should be made to lick a pinch of this powder mixed with a little honey. If need be, this should be fed on an hourly basis.

- Similarly, a peacock feather is burnt, charred and powdered and used in a manner as described above.

- Saunf ("Somp") is powdered and a spoon of this is dissolved in half a cup of hot water. The solution is allowed to stand till the particles settle at the bottom. The clear fluid on top of the sediment should be fed to the infant at the rate of one spoon per hour.

After feeding the infant it should be made to sit erect and its back gently massaged in a downward direction which prevents regurgitation and vomiting of the milk consumed. Water mixed with a pinch of salt and sugar is very effective in controlling vomiting in children of any age. In addition, the advice of a qualified paediatrician is essential.

LOOSE MOTION

Loose motion and consequent dehydration are common causes of infant mortality in case of an ill-developed immune system. The useful home-remedies are:

• Breast feeding should be immediately withheld and freshly prepared curd that has been fermented for four hours should be churned well and fed to the infant or child.

• Nutmeg should be ground in water and the paste thus obtained fed to the infant thrice daily. In case of severe loose motion with impending dehydration, this medicine should be given on an hourly basis.

• The skin of a pomegranate fruit is peeled off and crushed well. One spoon measure of this crushed skin is added to a cup of water and the mixture brought to boil. The medicinal solution or decoction thus obtained is decanted and fed to the infant at the rate of one spoon every hour.

• Nutgrass tubers are ground in honey to obtain a paste that is fed to the infant three times a day.

A solution of water and a pinch of salt and sugar is also effective against loose motion. But the advice of a qualified paediatrician is a must.

CONSTIPATION

It is common practice to feed an infant suffering from constipation with castor oil. This is very deleterious to the health of the child and at times even fatal. Castor oil irritates the colon of the infant and may cause severe diarrhoea. Hence, the following home remedies are indispensible:

• Chebulic myloboron nut is ground well in water and the paste thus obtained is fed in quantities of a quarter spoon three times a day. This relieves constipation and abdominal distension and increases the child's appetite.

• A part of a betel leaf, is dipped in castor oil for a while and is then gently applied to the anal region of the child. This softens the anal region and restores bowel movements.

• Castor oil is applied to a betel-leaf which is mildly warmed over a low flame. The warmed leaf when applied over the child's abdomen relieves the stomach ache and abdominal distension and restores bowel movements.

• Dry fig is squeezed in half a cup of water. This water is spoon fed very frequently. Similarly, sweet-lime juice is very effective in case of constipation in children.

ORAL ULCERS

If a lactating mother does not cleanse her nipples and the surrounding region of areola of her breast prior to feeding, there is every possibility of the infant developing oral ulcers. Hence, hygiene of the breast is of utmost importance in lactating mothers.

The simple home remedies that cure oral ulcers are:

• Pure honey when smeared frequently upon the ulcerated areas cures oral ulcers.

• The pulp in the core of a mango seed is extracted and ground well in pure honey. The paste thus obtained is fed to the infant three times a day.

• Coriander seeds are powdered and filtered over a clean piece of cloth. A pinch of this powder when sprinkled over the ulcerated areas cures them completely.

• The bark of the peepal tree is ground in pure honey and a paste is obtained. A quarter spoon of paste is fed three times a day to cure oral ulcers.

COUGH AND COLD

Cough and cold are the commonest enemies of a healthy child. They can strike at any moment and are prevalent throughout the year. The vulnerability of the infant's immune system and the varieties of common cold viruses are the main causes behind the recurrence of common cold.

The useful home remedies are:

• A pinch of powdered turmeric dissolved in a teaspoon of warm milk is fed tc the infant three times a day.

• Acorus plant is ground in water and the paste thus obtained is warmed over a low flame. The warm paste when applied as a pack over the forehead relieves the headache and nasal block associated with a bout of severe cold.

• A whole garlic is crushed well to extract the juice. A quarter spoon of juice mixed with equal quantity of pure honey is fed to the infant.

• Acorus is ground in water and a quarter spoon of the paste thus obtained is fed on an empty stomach followed by a cup of milk. This induces vomiting which immediately relieves symptoms of cold and cough.

• A few leaves of *tulasi*, thick leaved lavender and ruta are warmed (pre-heated) in an iron-pan over a low flame. The warmed leaves are then crushed to extract the juice. Quarter spoon of juice is fed thrice daily to cure common cold and cough.

• The flower of *vasaka* plant which grows abundantly in rural areas and is easily available for domestic use is crushed well to extract the juice. When this juice mixed with equal quantity of honey is fed to the infant frequently, the cough is immediately cured. In addition, the juice obtained by crushing the leaves of *vasaka* plant is very effective against cough in older children. One spoon of that juice should be taken three times a day.

NOCTURNAL ENEURESIS (BEDWETTING)

Some children suffer from bedwetting at night. Fear, lack of confidence and other psychological factors contribute a great deal to this disease. Proper counselling to ward off fear of any object is very essential to boost psychological health and prevent bedwetting.

The child must not go to bed until three hours have elapsed after dinner. Hence, an early dinner is preferable. Drinks that increase urine production such as fruit juice and milk must not be given at night.

Some helpful home remedies are:

• The roots of the little gourd creeper are crushed and the juice thus extracted is fed to the child just before going to bed.

• One spoon of finely powdered chebulic myloboron is added to half a cup of cold water early in the morning. The water floating on top of the sediment is given as a bed time drink to the child.

• Emblic myloboron is powdered well and filtered over a clean piece of cloth to separate the fine powder. Half a spoon of this powder mixed with honey is given to the child at bed time continuously for one whole week. This destroys the intestinal worms, increases appetite and relieves constipation as well as bedwetting.

Only some of the paediatric diseases responding to home remedies have been illustrated above. But a stitch in time saves nine. Hence, no disease should be neglected and allowed to take a violent course. A medicine once prescribed by a doctor must not be taken without medical consultation the next time similar symptoms are experienced. Nutritious food and hygiene are the building blocks of a child's health.

SPARSE HAIR AND DULL INTELLIGENCE IN CHILDREN:

Hair growth in children is completely determined by heredity and hence medicated oils should not be applied. A great deal of attention must be given to the child's health and nutrition. Care must be taken not to use very hot water when giving baths to children. Carrots are rich in Vitamin A and hence, one cup of carrot juice everyday makes a very healthy drink.

As the child grows, his bodily organs and the brain develop correspondingly. The I.Q. of a child increases with age.

Acorus is charred over a flame, ground well and honey added to it. A little quantity of this substance is mixed with pure ghee and given to the child early in the morning on an empty stomach say, on Wednesday and on the Sunday that comes immediately next.

Monthly blues of women

6

Women acquire sexual maturity between the ages of twelve and sixteen. The monthly cycle of menstruation that characterises female sexual maturity continues till the mid-forties when it finally comes to a halt. The book *Sushrutha Samhitha* gives a detailed description of the female reproductive system, the monthly menstruation cycle, the care of a pregnant woman and diseases affecting women.

Any change in the food habits and daily routine manifests itself as diseases in women. Among them, the following respond very well to home remedies:

WHITE DISCHARGE

This condition is an extremely common problem in women. It may also manifest itself as an adjunct to some other underlying disease. White discharge occurs for a few days after the normal menstrual cycle and also for some days before menstruation. At times, it may persist throughout the month leading to weakness, backache and the like, which require a specialist's care. Infections in the uterus and any other part of the female genital tract also causes white discharge. As prevention is always better than cure, regular exercise of the lower abdomen and rich, nutritious diet helps in the prevention of white discharge.

Some useful home remedies are as follows:

• A pinch of baking soda is added to a vessel containing lukewarm water and the resulting solution is used to clean the external genital organs three times a day.

Similarly an antiseptic solution prepared by heating neem leaves in water can be used to cleanse the genital organs. It destroys the bacteria growing in that part of the body.

• The water obtained after cleaning rice is filtered and one cup consumed thrice daily. This cures white discharge due to diseases of long standing. In addition, this water is a very rich source of vitamins that wards off weakness.

• The bark of red sandal is well ground in water to obtain a paste. Half a teaspoon of this paste is consumed early in the morning on an empty stomach followed by a cup of warm milk. Red sandal has cooling effect and it cures the pain and itching in the urinary and genital organs.

• A quarter spoon of lac stick powder is mixed with the requisite amount of honey and consumed twice daily. Half a cup of warm milk is consumed after this to find an effective cure.

DYSMENORRHOEA (*RUTHU SHOOLA*):

The first day of a menstrual cycle is associated with a pain in the lower abdomen. In addition, one is prone to vomiting, back ache and pain in the legs. This condition occurs very frequently in young women of marriageable age.

The useful home remedies for this condition are:

• Pieces of bark of the *Ashoka* tree are dried in sunlight. (Dried pieces are available readily in Pansari shops.) The dried bark is powdered well and one spoon of powder is added to a vessel holding three cups of water. The mixture is brought to boil and the vapours are allowed to escape till the resultant solution measures up to one cup. This solution is decanted and consumed three times a day. This regularises the menstrual cycle and also cures the pain. The term *Ashoka* is derived from its quality to cure pain. (*Shoka* means Pain in Sanskrit).

• Ruta leaves are dried in shade and ground into a fine powder. Quarter spoon of this powder mixed with equal quantity of sugar should be consumed three times a day.

• Leaves of the dead nettle white plant are cleansed in running water and crushed to extract the juice. One spoon of the juice is mixed with an equal quantity of lime juice and a pinch of common salt added. The resultant mixture is consumed three times a day throughout the period of menstruation (Average 3-5 days.)

• Gingiley oil is gently massaged over the lower abdomen, back and the upper thighs and left for a while. Later a hot water bath is taken to scrub the oil away. This procedure is extremely beneficial when done on a daily basis.

It is very interesting to note that skipping and dance are very important physical exercises that prevent dysmenorrhoea.

MENORRHAGIA OR EXCESSIVE MENSTRUATION

Some women experience excessive menstrual flow and the cycle occurs for a prolonged period. (Normal period is 3-5 days in a month). This leads to considerable loss of blood and resultant anaemia and weakness with genital and urinary tract infections. There are several causes of menorrhagia. Notable among these are infections in the uterus, congestion in the uterus and uterine fibroids. Hence a thorough gynaecological examination by an expert is very essential. When there are no physical defects in the uterus, only then can the following home remedies be used:

1. One handful of bermuda grass is washed in running water and added to a vessel holding

three cups of water. This is then brought to boil over a low flame till the volume is reduced to half. This solution is decanted and consumed three times a day. In addition to the cooling property, this grass also has a styptic effect (i.e. it arrests bleeding).

2. White clay is ground in milk and the paste thus obtained is consumed three times a day followed by a cup of cold milk.

3. Pieces of bark of the country fig are crushed well to obtain a powder. One spoon of this powder dissolved in a whole cup of milk is consumed three times a day.

4. The leaves of the "touch-me-not" plant are cleansed in running water and crushed to extract the juice. A piece of clean cotton is dipped in this extract and kept in close contact with the external genital and urinary organs like a sanitary pad. This takes care of infection and bleeding due to its antiseptic and styptic properties.

OLIGOMENORRHEA OR DEFICIENT MENSTRUATION:

Some women suffer from deficient menstrual blood flow inspite of regular menstrual cycles. This condition occurs due to several reasons but prime among these is anaemia which is very rampant in India. This is mainly due to illiteracy, poor nutrition and ignorance about health and hygiene.

The following home remedies offer fantastic results:

• Clean, dry cotton is burnt and the substance thus obtained is mixed with honey and consumed three times a day.

• Aloe is crushed to extract the juice. Three spoons of the juice are consumed three times a day.

• Asparagus is cleansed and crushed well to extract the juice. Two spoons of the juice mixed with half a cup of milk is consumed three times a day. This root even forms a nutritive supplement in all forms of diseases in women. This even enhances breast-milk in lactating mothers. *Sthreehi Rakshathi Rakshitha* is a popular saying from Ayurvedic texts. It implies that if the health of women is taken care of, her whole family is protected.

UNWANTED HAIR

Women commonly experience embarrassment due to excessive growth of hair in the wrong places viz. over the face, hands and legs. The problem is cosmetic but it also assumes psychosocial proportions. Hence, in olden days it was a common practice to use turmeric paste while taking off unwanted hair.

Since the above condition can also result from hormonal imbalances, a thorough examination by a qualified physician is essential. Only when no hormonal variations are detected, the following home remedies can be used:

• Turmeric, Indian barberry and round zedoary are taken in equal quantities and powdered well. This is mixed with green gram flour that is taken four times the quantity of the powder mixture. This is mixed with water and gently smeared on the areas of growth of unwanted hair. After a while, bath is taken in lukewarm water.

• The fruit of the acasia tree is broken to obtain the seed. The seed is then ground in water to obtain a paste which is smeared on the areas of unwanted hair. After a while, a lukewarm water bath is taken.

7

Wounds and injuries

In Ayurveda, *Vrana* is the term for all types of wounds. *Vrana Vastuna Nashyathi* – So states our Ayurvedic texts. This means that a wound makes its presence felt for a long time, in many cases it leaves behind a scar. Small wounds often respond remarkably to simple home remedies. But in case of large wounds, extensive areas of skin and flesh are left dead, which then have to be cut off and the ends sutured by qualified doctors. Patients suffering from varicose-veins i.e. enlarged veins in the thighs and legs often develop ulcerated wounds on the inner side of the lower leg. Likewise, diabetic patients develop similar wounds on the sole of the foot. These diabetic wounds tend to get infected very easily as the bacteria thrive in them due to the high glucose content in the blood supplying that area. If left untreated at the appropriate time, amputation of the limb may be necessary. These types of serious wounds are described as *Dushta Vrana* in Ayurveda (Dushta means wicked). It has also been stressed that these wounds have to be treated only by a qualified doctor.

Certain important guidelines need to be followed while treating minor injuries. Medicine should not be applied immediately on injuries sustained due to a fall as the wound would be teeming with bacteria. Hence, a thorough wash with ordinary soap and running water immediately, makes an excellent first-aid. Only then, should an antiseptic lotion be applied. In olden days, neem juice decoction was used for cleaning wounds due to its antiseptic properties. This destroys all the bacteria and ensures a speedy healing of the wound. In addition, three tablespoons of table salt should be dissolved in one small tumbler of lukewarm water and used to clean the wound. A solution of common salt also has great cleansing and healing properties.

OLD WOUNDS

Suppuration or pus formation is inevitable in old wounds because of bacterial infection. Prevention of pus accumulation is of utmost importance both for healing and for reducing scar formation. *Panchavalkala* is the name of the solution that works its magic in such cases. This is prepared by powdering the bark of five trees (Pancha means five in Sanskrit) viz. banyan, peepal, country fig, white fig and malbar tamarind and dissolving this powder in clean lukewarm water.

Nails should be trimmed as scratching with long nails not only hinders the healing process, but also introduces infection and worsens the wound.

The simple home remedies that are useful in treating wounds are:

• Tridax plant is washed well in running water. The leaves of the plant are separated, crushed and ground well and applied all over the wound. This immediately arrests the bleeding and facilitates speedy healing. This medicine also works wonders in healing wounds incurred while extracting a tooth.

• "Touch-me-not" plant is thoroughly washed, crushed and applied to the wound. This has both antiseptic and styptic (stoppage of bleeding) properties.

• Seven petalled jasmine plant is thoroughly washed and its leaves are separated. These leaves are ground well and applied all over the wound. This speeds the healing of wounds.

• Marigold plant is washed thoroughly and the leaves extracted. The crushed leaves of this plant have antiseptic properties. They reduce the pain in the wound and also prevent infection.

• The juice extracted from crushed green grass reduces itching, pain and bleeding in the wound.

• One spoon of glycyrrhiza powder is mixed with pure ghee and fried in a pan over a low flame. The paste thus obtained is slowly poured over the wound to reduce the pain.

• A requisite quantity of bee wax is taken and heated in a pan. The bee wax melts on application of heat, after which a little coconut oil is added to it and stirred well. The whole mixture is heated over a low flame, till it assumes a thick consistency. Later, the mixture is left to cool. The end result is a paste which is an excellent ointment for tough wounds. The ointment has proved its effectiveness for four generations.

LOCAL APPLICATIONS (LA):

In ancient times, leaves with medicinal properties were applied over the wounds. Three different types of local application of medicinal leaves are described in Ayurveda.

- The local application of a mixture of medicinal leaves in a thin layer, without pre-heating, is termed *Pralepa*.

- Similarly, the local application of a pre-heated mixture of medicinal leaves in a thick layer is termed *Pradheha*.

- Finally, the local application of a mixture of medicinal leaves heated to body temperature and applied in a medium sized layer is termed *Alepa* in Ayurveda.

It is extremely important to note that the local application has to be in a direction opposite to that of hair growth around the wound site. This enhances the healing properties of the medicine. After the medicine dries, it should be washed off before the layer withers away voluntarily and a new layer should be applied. This ensures sustained action of the medicine at the wound site and promotes healing. It also reduces scar formation.

In olden days when cotton bandages were not available, the wounds were bandaged using animal hides, raw skin, leaves and slender bark of trees. Even in the present day, betel leaves and plantain leaves are placed over the raw area of the wound and bandaged. Ayurveda states that closure of the wound using bandages is a must to prevent contamination and subsequent maggot infestation associated with severe infections. Hence, bandages act as a barrier between the raw surface of the wound and the external environment. In addition, antiseptic and pain killing sprays can also be used.

It is interesting to note that wounds heal slowly in winter and hence bandages need to be changed once every three days. During summer months, the healing process is fast and hence a daily change of bandages is mandatory.

Studies have revealed that food consumed has a great influence on the healing of wounds. Foods containing black gram, green peas, horsegram, beans, jaggery and curd should not be consumed during the healing period. Old stored rice, green leafy vegetables like celosia, orach, slender radish, brinjal, snake-gourd, bitter-gourd and pomegranate fruit are food that expedite the healing of wounds.

BURNS AND SCALDS

Burns are a universal phenomenon and they occur mostly in the kitchen. They are also common during Diwali. They are purely accidental, but at times they may be suicidal or homicidal, leading to medicolegal complications. It is important to learn some handy home remedies in the event of a burn injury.

• The water that remains in the vessel after washing rice, can be used to clean burn wounds occurring because of direct contact with fire. The wound is then gently wiped dry using a very clean cloth. This water prevents boils and reduces pain at the site of burn injury.

• A potato is washed well in running water and its skin peeled off. This skin is gently placed over the raw area of burn wounds and the whole area covered up. The wound is then bandaged firmly with the potato skin in place. This treatment immediately reduces pain and burning sensation and minimises scar formation.

• Local application of pure honey over the burn kills the bacteria owing to its antiseptic properties and promotes healing.

• Red sandalwood pieces are ground, mixed with water and the paste applied to the wound.

• Barley rice is burnt and the soot thus obtained is mixed in coconut oil to make a paste, which is applied to the burn.

• Ash gourd juice is sprinkled over the burn.

• One spoon of common salt and a pinch of baking soda are added to a vessel of water and stirred well. The solution is poured over the wound.

• Coconut water and a diluted solution of limestone or a little limestone paste itself can be gently applied over the burn as a pack.

• Til seeds and cow's milk are mixed in requisite quantities and ground. The mixture is applied to burn wounds sustained due to contact with moist heat like boiling water, oil, etc.

• Banana is crushed well and applied over the burns.

• A little common salt and pure ghee are mixed thoroughly to make a paste. This is applied to burns which are red and not accompanied by boils or exfoliation of skin.

All these home remedies are useful only in cases of minor burn wounds. In case of serious burns immediate medical attention is mandatory.

Like a shadow following us on a sunny day, a scar always follows a wound. With beauty conciousness on the rise, a scar is something to worry about. Additional expenses in the form of plastic surgery soon follow. As early as three thousand years ago, the sage Sushrutha, regarded as the "Father of Surgery", had devised a sur-

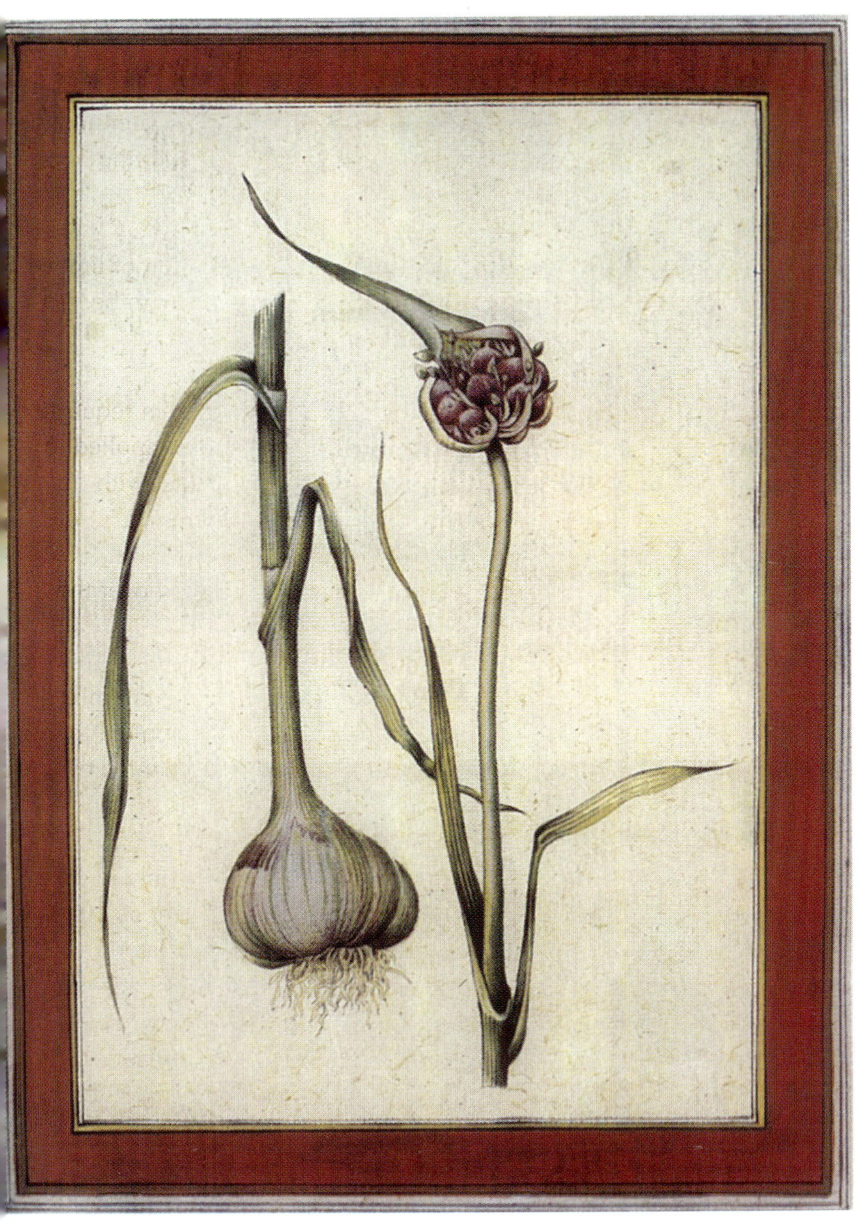

Garlic

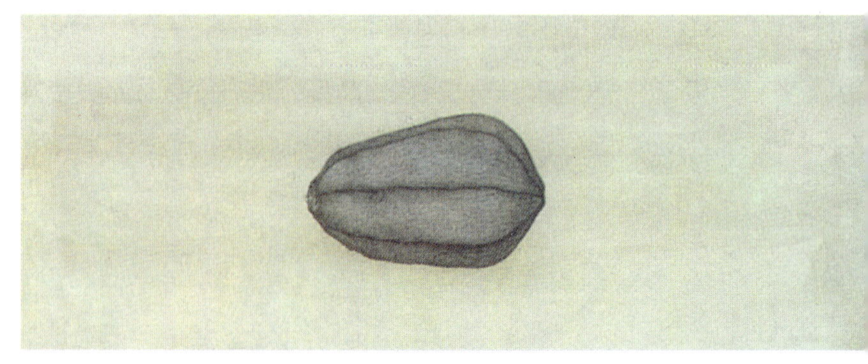

Chebulic Myrobalan

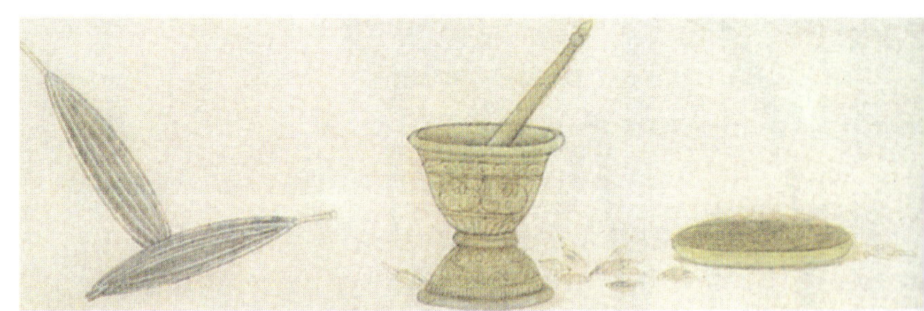

Cumin

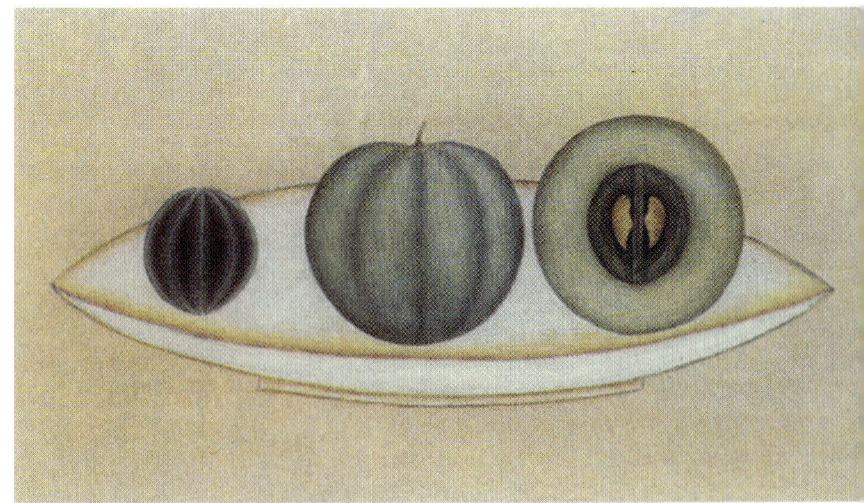

Emblic Myrobalan

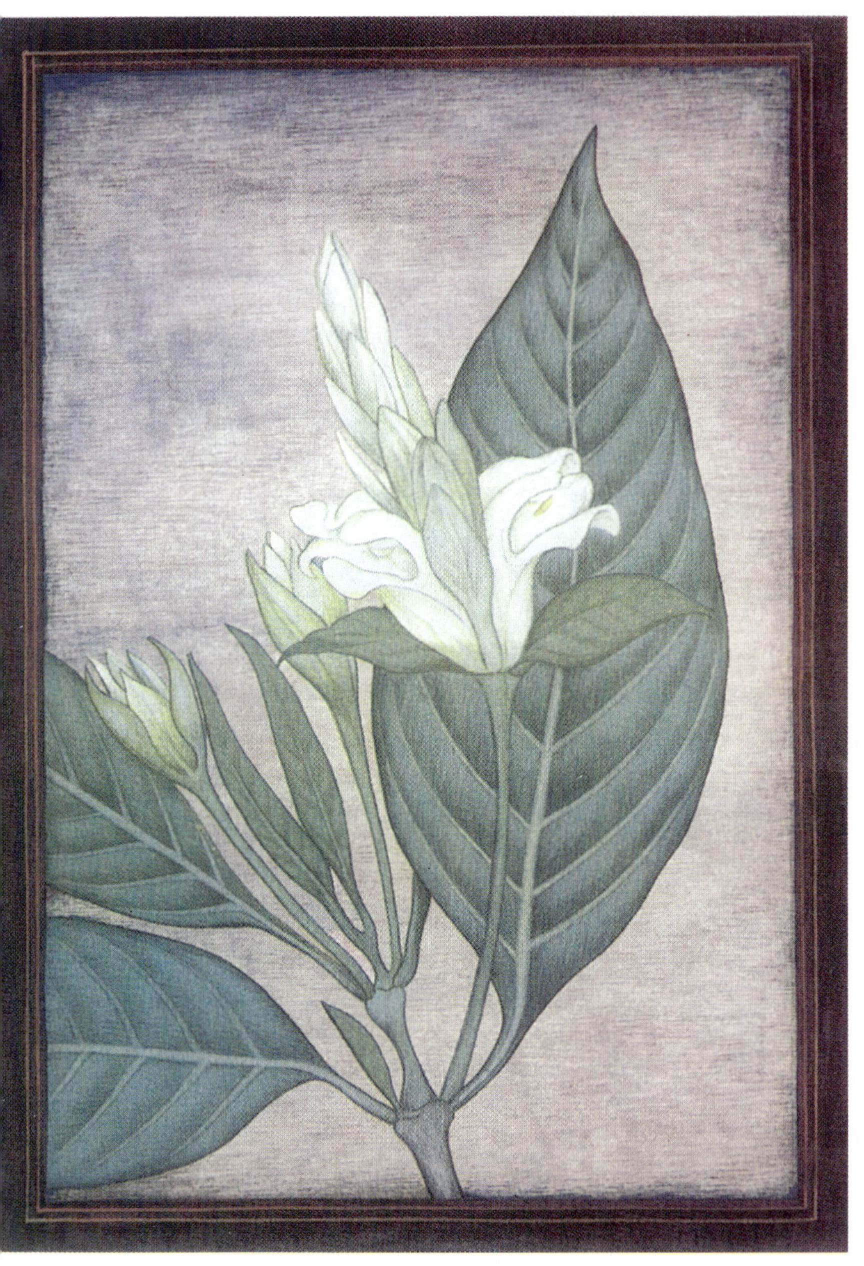

Vasaka

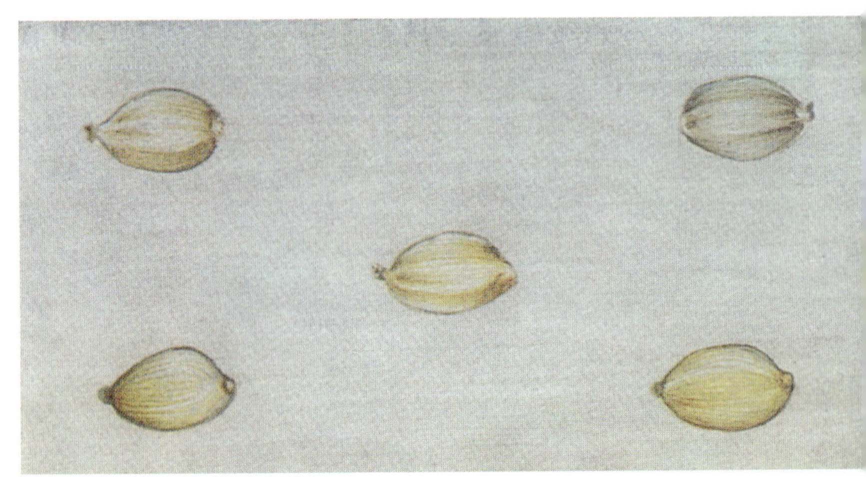

Cardamom

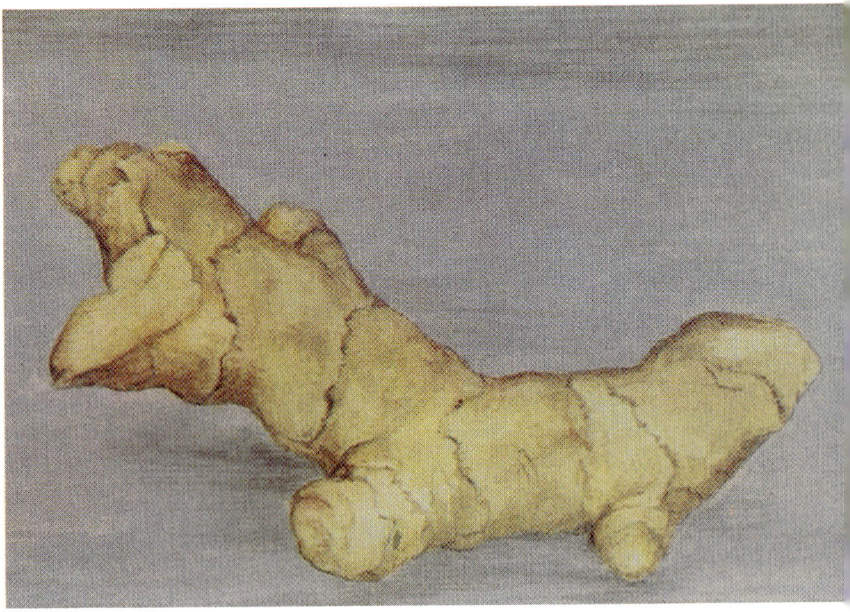

Ginger

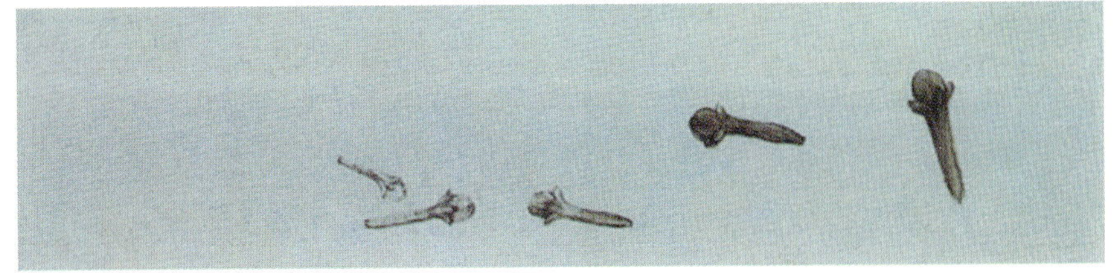

Clove

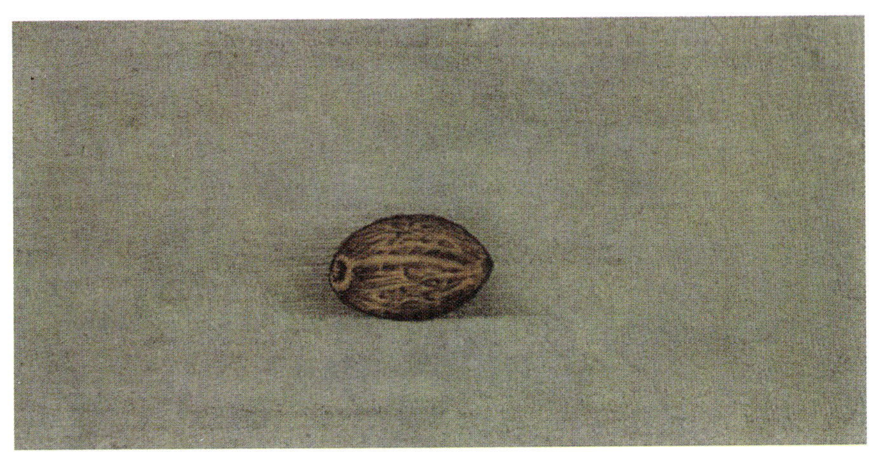

Nutmeg

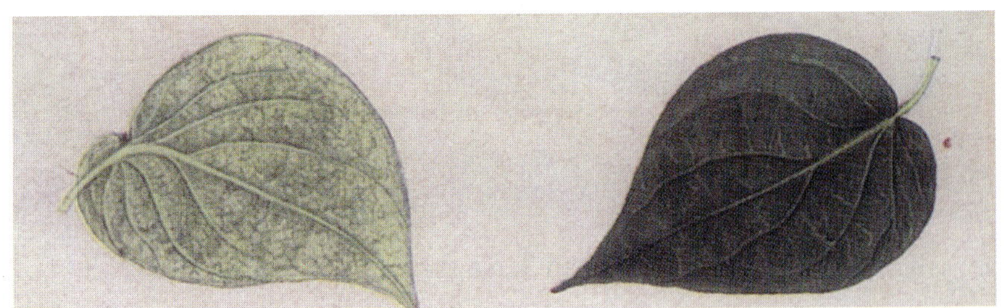

Betel Leaf

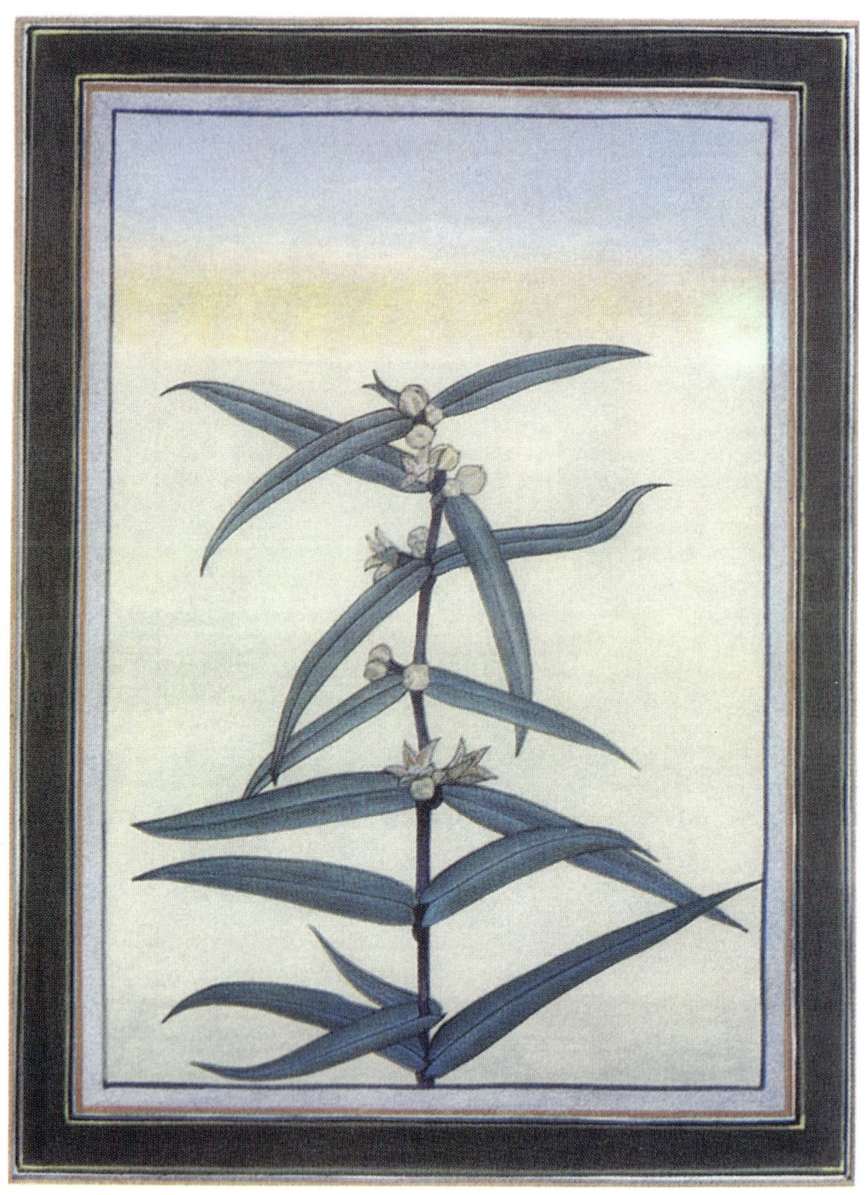

Indian Sarsa Parilla

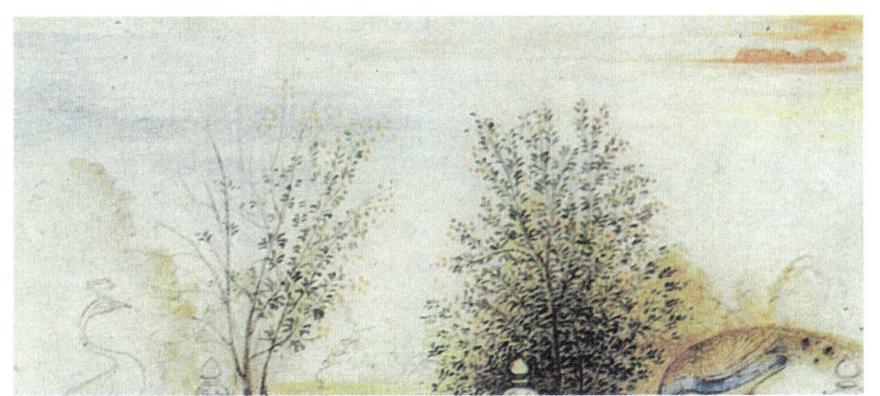

Henna

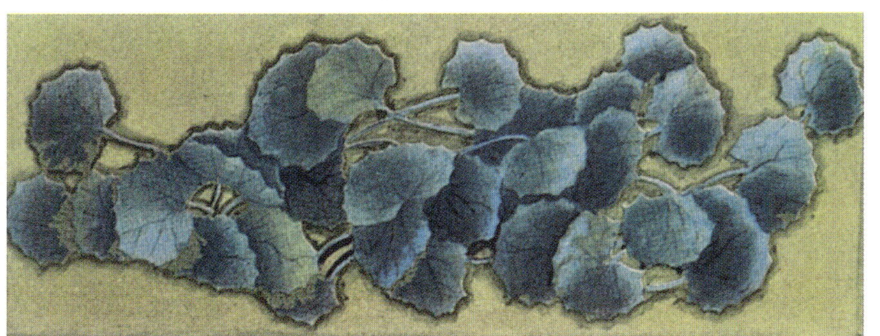

Indian Pennywort

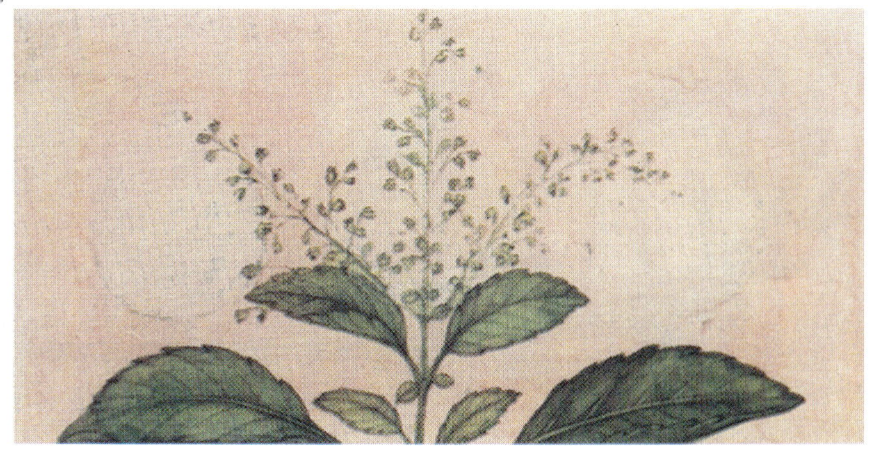

Basil

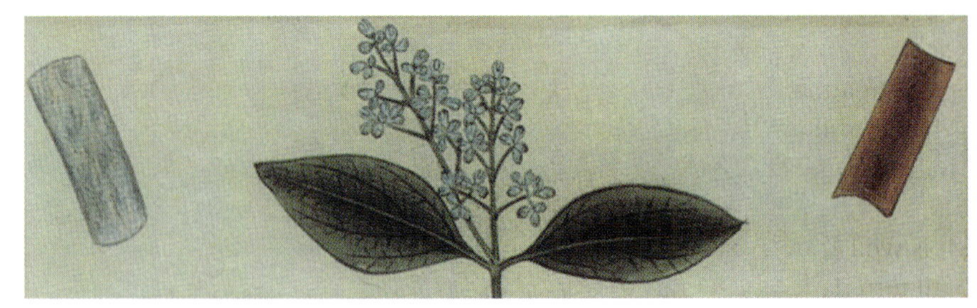

Cinnamon

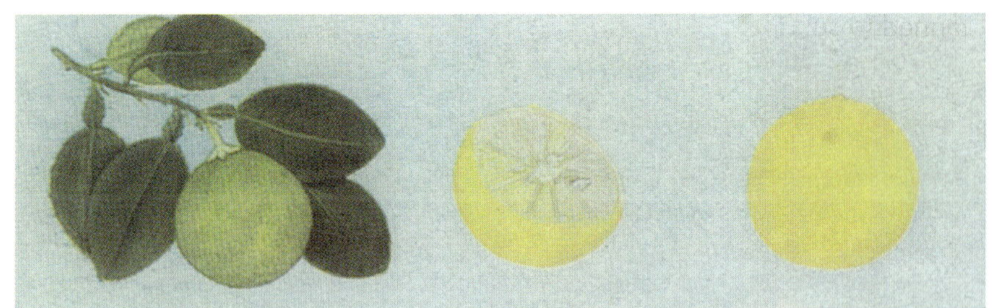

Lime

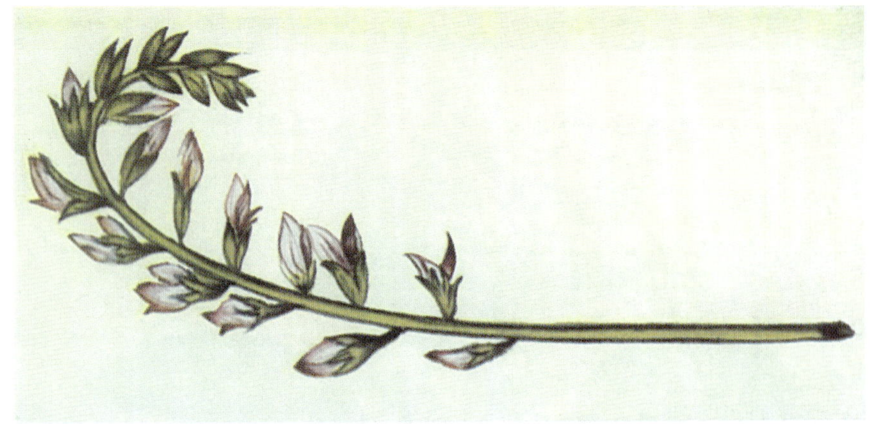

Liqvorice

gical treatment for scars called *Savarnikarana*. This term literally means restoration of the normal complexion to burnt skin.

It is well known that wounds sustained due to a fall turn dark on healing. This is treated by a technique called *Pandukarma* in which the dark colour of the skin is bleached to a fairer complexion. Burns on the other hand turn light (white) in colour on healing. This is treated by a technique called *Krishni-Karma* in which the affected skin is tanned to suit the body complexion.

8

Mother of all diseases - Indigestion!

Our ancestors termed fire as *Agni* in Sanskrit and recognised its presence in the human body. They justified that this *Agni* was present in the human body in the form of the digestive power of our digestive system, the special senses of the eyes, ears, nose, tongue and skin, the warmth of body-temperature and finally in the form of skin complexion and muscle power. *Agni* was also synonymously termed *Pittha*, stated to be present in each and every cell of the human body but predominantly in the centre of the stomach and small intestine, according to Ayurveda. This *Pittha* functions in the body in the form of bile secreted by the liver and insulin secreted by the pancreas.

Increased frequency of meals, untimely meals, junk food, lack of exercise and above all rising levels of mental stress work in coalition to put the digestive powers out of gear. In common parlance, this means that the above causes lead to imbalance in digestion or indigestion. This is termed *Agnimandhya* in Ayurveda and has been described as "the mother of all diseases". This condition leads to lack of taste and appetite.

POOR DIGESTION (*AMAJEERNA*)

Excessive and untimely consumption of junk food and aerated cool drinks result in weakened digestive powers and indigestion. The whole symptom complex associated with the above condition is termed *Amajeerna* in Ayurveda. This condition manifests itself as stomach upsets, obesity, headache and increased salivation which are accompanied by symptoms of common cold, cough, fever and sputum production.

The useful home remedies for this conditions are:

• Saunf seeds are powdered. Half a spoon of this powder is dissolved in a cup of water and consumed three times a day. These seeds have the property of increasing appetite termed as *Deepana* and they also enhance taste.

• Fresh ginger is crushed well to extract its juice. An equal quantity of honey is mixed with the juice and consumed frequently.

• Dry ginger is powdered. Quarter teaspoon of the powder is mixed with equal quantity of powdered jaggery and consumed three times a day.

• Dry ginger is cut into small pieces and rinsed in lime juice extract and a little common salt. Three pieces are later dried in sunlight. These pieces are then kept in the sides of the mouth and their juice sucked. This medicine restores taste sensation.

• Nagkeshar stamens is powdered and half a spoon of powder mixed with pure ghee is consumed three times a day. This restores normal digestive powers and appetite, thus relieving even indigestion due to long standing disease. Ginger and Nagkeshar stamens are termed *Pachaka* due to their digestive properties.

But prevention is always better than cure. The preventive measures against indigestion are:

• Frequent consumption of hot water.

• Consumption of light food and avoiding over-eating.

• Preference for fluid diet as against solid diet.

• Regular physical exercise

Indigestion surely becomes a thing of the past when these measures are strictly followed.

EXCESSIVE HUNGER AND INDIGESTION (*VIDAGDHAJEERNA*)

Excessive consumption of spice, hot and sour food stuffs and uncontrolled alcoholism cause indigestion and result in the condition termed as gastritis and consequently stomach ulcer. This condition is characterised by a burning sensation in the stomach, the centre of the chest and commonly the mouth and throat also.

The patient suffers from mouth ulcers, dizziness, nausea, excessive belching and burning sensation in the centre of the chest.

The home remedies that provide an effective cure are the following:

- Half a teaspoon each of cumin seeds and coriander seeds are added to half a cup of water taken in a vessel and the mixture is brought to boil. The solution is then decanted and consumed three times a day.

- Cumin seeds are powdered well and half a teaspoon of powder mixed with equal quantity of jaggery powder is consumed twice daily after meals.

- Dry gooseberry is powdered and half a teaspoon of powder mixed with equal quantity of sugar is consumed three times a day.

- Liquorice is powdered and half a spoon of this powder dissolved in a quarter cup of fresh cow's milk is consumed twice daily.

Drinking a bellyful of water on an empty stomach and using ash gourd and bottle gourd in the daily diet are some of the preventive measures for gastritis.

ERRATIC DIGESTION (*VISHTAMBHAJEERNA*)

Another important form of indigestion is erratic digestion which occurs due to the following faults in lifestyle:

- Curbing hunger and going on an empty stomach very often.

• Prolonged interval between meals and untimely food habits.

• Excessive consumption of coffee, tea or any beverage containing cocoa.

• Chain-smoking.

• Inadequate hours of sleep.

• Above all, mental stress which is a part and parcel of urban life.

This condition presents itself with the symptoms of stomach discomfort, excessive belching, stomach ache, headache and constipation.

The preventive measures against this condition are
• Adequate bed rest.

• Frequent consumption of hot milk in small doses

• Having oil bath at least twice or thrice a week.

• Inclusion of gruel and sweet gruel in the diet.

The useful home remedies for this condition are:
• Pure asafoetida with a little ghee added, is fried in a pan. A pinch of this fried asafoetida is added to a morsel of cooked rice and a little common salt is sprinkled. The morsel is consumed before taking a meal.

• Dry-ginger, pepper, long pepper, saunf, rocksalt, cumin seeds and black cumin seeds are taken in equal quantities and powdered. The powder is then filtered to obtain the fine powder. Pure asaoetida is taken in 1/7th the quantity of the above and fried in ghee. This is added to the fine powder mixture. The ultimate mixture gets the name *Hingwashtaka churna* which is extremely useful in any type of indigestion. Half a teaspoon of this powder is mixed with one morselful of rice and consumed as medicine. Also, consumption of churned butter milk mixed with the *Hingwashtaka* powder relieves stomach discomfort, gas and loose motions. If this powder is consumed along with hot water, it arrests belching and increases appetite.

• Garlic is peeled and the vegetable cut into small pieces. The pieces are fried in pure ghee, mixed with steamed rice and consumed.

As stated previously, Ayurveda regards indigestion as the "mother of all diseases" and hence treatment of indigestion should always be the first step in curing any disease, big, small or chronic.

9 Headache

Any pain in the head is referred to as a headache irrespective of the area it affects, except for the organs of special senses. As no man on earth is untouched by headache, the market is flooded with medicines that promise to cure this universal problem. According to a wise saying, it is foolish to take the same type of medicine for any type of headache. For example if the pain is present in between the eyebrows, the central part of the forehead and both sides of the nose, it is headache due to common cold.

The useful home remedies for the above conditions are:

• Dry ginger powder is mixed with requisite amount of water to a paste-like consistency. The paste is then slightly warmed and applied as a pack over the forehead. This treatment melts the thickened mucus which is blown out of the nose at regular intervals and hence relieves headache. In addition, the warmth of the medicine increases the local blood circulation which also helps to relieve pain.

• To a tumbler of boiling water, one spoonful of eucalyptus oil is added and the emerging vapour taken in by deep inhalation. The eucalyptus vapours melt the inspissated mucus to relieve the headache.

• Half a spoon of black pepper is powdered and added to half a cup of warm milk. A little jaggery powder (not sugar) is added to taste and the milk is consumed three times a day. This not only relieves the congestion in the nose and throat but also cures indigestion and increases appetite.

• Kulijan, cumin seeds, coriander seeds and dry ginger are taken in equal quantities and powdered. One spoon of the powder is added to a tumbler containing two cups of water and the solution is brought to boil till it vapourises to half its previous volume. The final solution is decanted and consumed thrice daily. This medicine cures headache, body ache and fever. Headaches arising from exposure to cold can be prevented by avoiding exercise or walking in a cold environment. Deep inhalation of cold, moist air increases mucus secretion that clog the sinuses in the forehead and the sides of the nose, leading to heaviness and aching sensation in the head. Consumption of chilled drinks after physical exertion in hot climates also leads to immediate headache in susceptible individuals. Such habits should be given up.

A pain in the eyes and the back of the head is common among students and in those whose work involves long hours of reading and concentrated study. This occurs due to refractive errors in the eyes and needs an opthalmologist's (eye-specialist) opinion, in addition to the following home remedies:

• Sandalwood is ground in water to obtain the paste. Two pieces of cotton are dipped in clean water, squeezed to remove excess water and then smeared with the sandal paste. These cotton pieces are placed, one on each eyelid while going to bed. This provides a cooling effect and relieves the headache due to refractive errors of the eye. Alternately, white clay can be ground in water and its paste smeared over the eyelids before going to bed to obtain similar relief.

• There is a popular saying which states that alternanthera restores vision even to blind eyes. This green leafy vegetable is a rich source of Vitamin A, similar to carrot, and when consumed on a regular basis, relieves headache due to eye problems.

• Home made eyeliner prepared from flowers of nerium plant or alternanthera plant or from white onion is applied to the eyelids at night. It is always safe and hygienic to use home made eyeliners.

The following are some valuable tips to prevent headaches due to eye problems:

• Long hours of reading, study or watching T.V. without regular breaks, should be avoided.

• Reading in dim light should be avoided.

• Reading in lying down position should be avoided.

All the above activities, cause strain to the eyes which in turn leads to a headache.

MIGRAINE

An excrutiating pain on either sides of the forehead that is alleviated after a bout of vomiting is termed as migraine attack or simply migraine headache. Though the exact cause of this condition remains uncertain, acidity in the stomach and sudden episodic enlargement of the blood vessels supplying the head have been recognised as causes. Rising levels of stress in daily life, untimely meals, consumption of coffee or tea very often are some of the causes attributed to migraine. High levels of caffeine in coffee irritate the stomach causing acidity and it also enters the blood causing episodic enlargement of blood vessels. Migraine attacks can be prevented by following these guidelines:

• Timely food habits.

• Occasional consumption of tea or coffee.

• Consumption of a cup of cold water before having coffee or tea.

Inadequate water consumption and excess spice in the diet also increase acidity and hence have to be given up.

It is advisable to learn by heart and follow this saying:

"Drink like a fish, but, drink what fish drinks".

The following home remedies drive out migraine:

• Half a spoon each of coriander seeds and cumin seeds are powdered, added to a tumbler holding a cup of water and boiled. The solution is then decanted and half a cup of milk and a little sugar to taste are added. This medicine when consumed two to three times a day provides an efficient cure for migraine and also decreases the acidity in the stomach.

• A drop of pure ghee is added to each nostril and deep breathing is practised closing one nostril at a time. This rests the nerves in the forehead and hence relieves headache.

• An onion is crushed to extract the juice. Two spoons of this juice is mixed with an equal quantity of pure honey and consumed once in the morning and once at night. Diabetic patients should not use honey. Consumption of this medicine leaves a pungent odour in the mouth and it should be followed by mouth wash and throat gargling. Onion brings down stomach acidity and relieves the headache.

• Mustard is well ground in water and warmed over a low flame. This is then applied as a pack over the forehead to get rid of the headache.

A nagging pain in the neck and head is an invariable by-product of prolonged hours of office-work with the neck bent. The ache in the head and neck occurs due to strain on the nerves of the neck. Hence, slow forward and backward bending exercises of the neck have to be done regularly.

The home remedies that tackle the above condition are as follows:

• Mustard oil is gently massaged starting from the back of the ear, down the neck, to the shoulder upto the upper arm. The massage should again start from the back of the ear and the massaging hand should not be brought back in the reverse direction after one round of massage. Mustard oil increases the local blood circulation in the muscles and relieves muscular-spasm and pain.

• It is believed that ruta plant keeps snakes away due to the peculiar scent that it gives off. A handful of ruta leaves are taken and crushed well. One cup of olive oil is boiled in a vessel, the crushed leaves are slowly added to it and the vessel is closed. After the oil cools down, it is decanted and used to massage the neck from above downwards to relieve the pain. This oil also relieves the pain in the forehead occurring due to common cold.

• The white flowers of the *dhatura* plant bear a close resemblance to the old gramaphone speaker. The leaves of this plant are washed in running water and crushed thoroughly. A hot, concentrated solution of powdered jaggery is prepared and the crushed leaves are added to it. After thorough cooling, the mixture assumes the consistency of an ointment. This ointment is applied to the forehead and neck to relieve the pain. A headache occuring due to an infection in the brain or its covering or a tumour growing in the brain have to be thoroughly investigated and treated only by a neuro specialist. Hence, negligence of a chronic headache is extremely unwise.

Hairfall and dandruff

10

The palms, soles and the lips are the only parts of the body that are spared of hair growth. In animals, hair conserves body temperature, but in human beings, hair on the head adds to physical beauty and at the same time acts as a protective covering . Ancient texts estimate that there are around one lakh hairs on the scalp, of which 5-6 old ones fall off each day and new ones take birth simultaneously. The inner layer of the skin called dermis houses the roots of hairs. As wrinkles in the skin mark the dawn of ageing process, so does hairfall. But, hairfall in the young assumes cosmetic importance and occurs due to the following reasons:

• Influence of heredity when the parents have sparse hair.

• Infrequent head bath due to negligence of cleanliness and hygiene. It is worthwhile to remember that "Cleanliness is next to Godliness".

• Malnutrition and lack of vitamins and minerals in the diet. This also leads to premature greying.

• Mental stress, worry and anxiety are also indirect causes.

It is a vicious cycle that increased worry leads to increased hairfall which in turn increases worry. The following home remedies arrest hairfall and promote hair growth:

• It is common to find a small plant growing by the roadside which resembles the flowers of Tridax. This plant is termed Eclipta or *Bhringaraja* in Sanskrit and grows in close proximity to water. *Bhringa* means "Drone" in Sanskrit and this plant also called *Bringharaja* helps in the growth of rich black hair that resemble the colour of drone. Leaves of this plant are crushed and the juice extracted. To this juice is added double its volume of olive oil or coconut oil and is brought to boil. After the water content evaporates, the oil is left to cool and gently massaged into the scalp.

• Similarly, henna leaves that are used to beautify hands and legs, are crushed, boiled in coconut oil and used as hair oil as stated above.

• Lime juice extract is gently massaged all over the scalp, left for an hour and then washed away. The citric acid in lime stimulates the hair roots and hence promotes hair growth. In addition, it also nourishes the hair.

• Leaves of hibiscus or white flower are ground and the juice extracted is mixed with double its volume of coconut oil and boiled. The hair oil thus prepared prevents hairfall and promotes hair growth.

• Indian pennywort is a small plant that grows in close affinity to water and is very popular as a memory booster. The leaf of this plant resembles a frog's face and hence it is termed *Mandookaparni* in Sanskrit. (Mandooka meaning frog). As leaves directly take origin from its slender stem, the plant is also termed Indian Pennywort. The whole plant including the leaves, stem and the roots, is carefully uprooted from the soil, washed thoroughly in running water and ground well. The juice extracted is mixed with double its volume of coconut oil and boiled. The resulting oil is cooled and used as hair oil to stop hair fall due to worry, anxiety and mental stress.

• Decanted and cooled tea decoction is a marvellous medicine which prevents hairfall if used to wash hair. This decoction has a hard taste and it decreases the oil secreted by the skin of the scalp, thereby promoting hair growth.

• Two spoons of powdered amla (dry gooseberry) are added to a tumbler holding two cups of water and boiled once. The resulting solution is cooled and used to wash hair during a head

bath. This medicine prevents hairfall and promotes hair growth. Similarly, if the above solution is mixed with double its quantity of coconut oil and boiled, the resultant hair oil also produces a beneficial effect on scalp hairs.
Gooseberry is rich in Vitamin 'C' which nourishes the hair roots.

• Likewise, alternanthera is washed in running water and crushed well. The juice thus extracted is mixed with double its quantity of coconut oil and boiled. The hair oil thus prepared promotes hair growth and nourishes the hair roots due to its abundant Vitamin 'A' content.
Frequent hair washes prevent hairfall as they promote hygiene. It is also advisable to use lukewarm water while taking a head bath because hot water weakens the hair roots and facilitates hairfall. Dandruff, lice-infestation, skin and hair infections spread from one person to another due to sharing of combs, towels, helmets etc. Hence, combs at least should never be shared. It is also noted that a cold water head bath increases blood circulation in the scalp and promotes hair growth.

A diet rich in sprouts, milk and raw carrots is very nutritious for the hair roots and promotes abundant hair growth. Increased sweating brought about by physical exercise also promotes hair growth.

DANDRUFF

Dandruff is a condition characterised by heat,

redness and itching of the scalp skin with subsequent scaling. The itching sensation increases by the day and the dry, scalp skin withers away as thin, white flakes. These flakes fall on the skin of the face giving rise to small pimple like eruptions. This condition occurs due to the growth of lice on the scalp skin. Hence, sharing combs or towels should be strictly avoided. In addition, one of the main causes of hairfall, such as anxiety and mental stress, is also a cause of dandruff.

Excessive consumption of fried and oily food also increases dandruff production.

The useful home remedies for dandruff are:

• Two teaspoons each of methi and cumin seeds are soaked overnight in a vessel with water that is just sufficient to hold them. The next morning, the mixture is ground and applied to the scalp. After half an hour, a head bath with lukewarm water is taken.

• One handful of methi leaves and two spoons of methi seeds are ground in milk and applied to the scalp. A head bath after half an hour relieves the dandruff and promotes hair growth. This medicine also relieves itching and prevents infection due to its antiseptic properties.

• The pulp of the mango seed is extracted and ground in milk. The paste thus obtained is applied to the scalp and left for half an hour. Later, a head bath is taken with lukewarm water.

• The skin of a dried lime fruit is powdered and

to this is added four times its quantity of green gram flour and mixed thoroughly. When this powder is frequently used to wash hair, it cures dandruff and prevents hairfall.

Incomplete drying of hair after a head bath facilitates an uncontrolled growth of fungus due to the moisture in the hair, thereby increasing dandruff. Hence, complete drying of hair after a head bath is a must. Improper capping of coconut oil bottles in cold weather promotes growth of fungus on the oil surface, which when applied to the hair causes dandruff.

HAIRLESS PATCHES OF SKIN ON THE SCALP AND FACE

This condition is termed *Indraluptha* in Ayurveda. Hairless patches gain cosmetic importance and hence their treatment is rewarding.

The home remedies that address this condition are:

- The hairless patch of skin is wet and gently scrubbed with a leaf of night jasmine tree. This procedure roughens the smooth skin surface of the hairless patch and stimulates hair growth.

- Bitter gourd leaves are crushed and the juice is applied to the hairless patch and gently massaged to promote hair growth.

- Indian liquorice is ground in lime juice extract and the paste is applied to the hairless patch.

11

Diseases of the teeth and mouth ulcers

A face lit up by dazzling smile is a welcome sight indeed. Undoubtedly, the dentures are responsible for the smile. In poetic parlance, well set dentures are compared to a pomegranate. According to a popular saying, the mouth is the index of the digestive system. Hence, dental hygiene tops the list of healthy habits.

The importance of dental hygiene is increasingly felt with advances in civilisation. Hence, a wide range of products are available for protection of dental health.

The following guidelines can go a long way in protecting dental health:

- Consumption of food that is either too hot or too cold weakens the dental roots and facilitates premature fall of teeth. For example frequent consumption of very hot coffee or tea, or very cold beverages, soft-drinks or ice-creams, loosen the roots of the teeth and at the same time create a thriving ground for bacteria due to their high sugar-content. Hence, these food items have to be consumed in limited quantities.

• As children naturally love chocolates, candies and sweets, excessive consumption of these food stuffs cause dental caries and toothache. Hence, it is advisable to train children to gargle and have a thorough mouth wash with warm water after eating chocolates or sweets. Warm water flushes out the food particles sedimented between the teeth, kills bacteria and prevents infections. This also prevents bad mouth odour.

• Excessive use of toothpicks to pick the spaces between the teeth after having food, weakens the roots of the dentures which fall off early. Hence, toothpicks should be minimally used.

• Though *paan* and *beeda* improve digestion they are injurious to dental health.

• The bacteria causing dental caries and mouth infections may be swallowed with food and hence cause infection of the digestive system or gastroenteritis which presents as vomiting, loose motions, fever and loss of appetite.

These bacteria commonly infect the tonsils in the throat leading to its infection called tonsillitis which presents as fever, pain in the throat on swallowing, difficulty in swallowing and mouth odour. These bacteria also cause sore throat and arthritis.

The common dental problems are toothache, mouth odour, bleeding gums, pain in the gums and dental caries. The simple and trustworthy home remedies for these conditions are described here:

TOOTHACHE

• Dried gooseberries are powdered and half a spoon of this powder is dissolved in a vessel holding two cups of water. The solution is boiled till it evaporates to half its previous volume and then cooled. This is used as a mouthwash three times a day.

• A handful of leaves of the guava tree are washed in running water and crushed well. The crushed leaves are added to a vessel holding two cups of water, boiled, cooled and then decanted. When the resultant solution is used as a mouthwash, toothache is relieved.

• Mango leaves can be used in a similar manner as the guava leaves and its solution used as a mouthwash. In addition to curing toothache, the above medicine also increases appetite and improves digestion.

• A mouthwash prepared from tender mango leaves has a stronger effect.

MOUTH ODOUR

The beauty of a picture perfect face is ruined by poor dental hygiene resulting in a foul odour from the mouth. The following home remedies hold promise:

• Basil leaves are chewed once in the day and once in the night to get rid of mouth odour all day long.

• One spoon of long-pepper powder is mixed with half a spoon of pure ghee and a quarter spoon of pure honey and the whole mixture is consumed two to three times a day. This medicine drives out mouth odour, strengthens the gums and improves digestion too.

• One handful of leaves of the pomegranate tree are crushed, added to a tumbler holding two cups of water, boiled, cooled and decanted. The final solution is used as a mouthwash to get rid of foul odour.

• Catechu is powdered and a quarter spoon of this powder is gently rubbed over the teeth and gums three times a day. After a while, the mouth is washed with lukewarm water.

BLEEDING GUMS

• A handful of leaves of the touch-me-not plant are washed in running water, crushed well, added to a tumbler holding two cups of water, boiled, cooled and then decanted. The resulting solution is used as a mouthwash three times a day to immediately stop bleeding in the gums. This is because the touch-me-not plant, as described elsewhere, is a styptic i.e., it has anti-bleeding properties.

• Arecanut is burnt till it is charred and later powdered. This powder is taken in small quantities at a time, mixed with equal quantity of common salt and used as a tooth powder while brushing teeth.

DENTAL CARIES

Though dental caries find a permanent cure only with a qualified dentist, the following home remedies can alleviate the pain associated with the condition.

• The seed of the jamboo fruit is dried, powdered and then burnt. The charred powder is then gently massaged over the carious tooth to lessen the suffering.

• A clove is powdered and held firmly against the carious tooth to get rid of the pain.

• A piece of turmeric is charred and powdered. This powder is mixed with equal quantity of common salt and used as a toothpowder. This relieves the pain in the carious tooth and at the same time prevents infection due to its antiseptic properties.

MOUTH ULCERS

An ulcer is defined as a break in the continuity of the skin or mucous-membrane i.e. any protective covering layer in the body in general. It is common to find ulcers resulting from scratching insect bites, skin infections, the lower leg ulcer in varicose (enlarged) leg-veins etc.

Similar, but smaller ulcers occur frequently on

the soft and slimy mucous membrane layer covering the inner aspect of the mouth. These ulcers are termed Oral ulcers or commonly Mouth-ulcers. The inner aspect and the margins of the upper and lower lip, the gums, the margins and either surface of the tongue and the inner aspect of the cheek in close contact with the dentures are the common sites for mouth ulcers. These ulcers may present as reddened, circular ones or as innumerable spotted ulcers. They cause pain while chewing and hence make eating food a painful experience. An ulcer at the margin of the tongue interferes with clear pronounciation of words.

Though there are several causes of mouth ulcers, chronic indigestion is the most prominent one. A friction with the teeth while chewing, improper ways of brushing teeth, wrong choice of tooth brush, an irritant tooth paste are other important causes of mouth ulcers. In addition, they also occur as a side effect of certain oral medicines. Poor hygiene of a mother's nipples, feeding the infant without washing the nipples, infection of the breasts and inadequate sterilisation of the feeding bottle are important causes of mouth ulcers among infants. A dietary deficiency of Vitamin B, Vitamin C and iron also causes mouth ulcers in infants and children. In adults, excessive smoking and alcoholism irritates the mucous membrane of the mouth causing ulcers. Diseases of the teeth and gums, acidity in the stomach, loose motion, indigestion and constipation also create mouth ulcers which are extremely painful. In addition, the ulcers due to stomach upset, acidity and excessive belching of foul air are accompanied by an intense burning sensation. Itching is a prominent feature of ulcers due to common-cold, cough and lung infections. The time tested home remedies for this distressing condition are:

- Good dental hygiene which includes brushing teeth twice a day keeps mouth ulcers away. A handful of bermuda grass is thoroughly washed in running water and crushed. This is added to a vessel holding two cups of water, boiled, cooled and finally decanted. The resulting solution when used as a mouth wash cures the mouth ulcers very fast.

- A small quantity of catechu is mixed with equal quantity of sugar candy. A pinch of this mixture is consumed twice a day. Also, a pinch of the same mixture is powdered and dissolved in half a cup of warm water and used as a mouthwash.

- Oak galls are well ground in water and the paste obtained is applied over the mouth ulcers to cure them.

- A warm decoction of tea leaves when used as a mouth wash two to three times a day is also very beneficial.

- Basella, a green leafy vegetable which is very rich in vitamin B must be an integral part of the daily diet to get rid of mouth ulcers.

• Five black coloured raisins are soaked in water and consumed twice daily after thorough chewing.

• Half a spoon of cumin seeds are powdered, added to half a cup of water in a vessel and boiled. After decantation, a little milk is added to the solution and consumed early in the morning on an empty stomach. These home remedies give long lasting relief from mouth ulcers and prevent their recurrence.

12

Teenage blues with pimples!

Pimples, literally, make the teenage population see red. Especially girls, when the mirror points out these daunting little things that spring up from nowhere on their faces. Pimples form a hot topic of discussion in any college-campus or teenage parties and gatherings. With beauty conciousness on the rise in the wake of our country producing international beauty queens year after year, these teenagers try moving heaven and earth to get rid of those pimples. These are a natural part of growing up after sexual maturity. Any effort against nature is futile and hence any attempt at uprooting pimples can only be desperate. Not only does this burn a huge hole in the pocket of the parents but also drives these teenagers into a frenzy. But the worst part is that this problem assumes great psychological implications and the affected teenager withdraws into himself to escape the teasing from his peers. Hence, pimples are not just skin disease but also have a deleterious effect on one's psychology. Awareness has to be generated among teenagers that pimples are an integral part of the growing up process and not anything unnatural.

The technical term for pimples is Acne Vulgaris. They are called *Youvvana Pidaka* in Sanskrit meaning "pustules in youth". A pustule is a small swelling in the skin filled with pus. The hormonal changes that occur in the body during sexual maturity trigger the onset of pimples. Excessive consumption of fried and oily food stuff, foods rich in cocoa like chocolates, candies etc., and sweets are also causes of Acne Vulgaris. Heredity is an extremely important causative factor. In girls, these pimples flare up around the period of menstruation. A frequent change in the brand of toilet soap used is also one of the causes. This is because the skin has a tendency to adapt itself to one kind of soap that suits it best.

A simple home made powder provides an efficient control for pimples. Red *toor dal*, rice grains, *jowar*, green peas and *channa dal* are all taken in equal quantities and powdered well. This powder is used as a face wash two to three times a day. This face wash completely clears the face off pimples and prevents scar formation too.

It is important to note that pimples appear more in oily skin. This is because, the oil secreted by the skin blocks the opening of the sweat glands on the skin, leading to accumulation of their secretion, subsequent infection and pustule formation. This eventually leads to pimples. Hence, the face should be kept oil free by washing with one adapted brand of soap two to three times a day. The market today is flooded with creams, lotions, face packs, face wash, soaps and blood-purifiers that promise to ward off pimples. These items are not only heavy on the wallet but also provide unsatisfactory results leaving the user frustrated. The following cost-effective, time-tested and safe home remedies provide an effective alternative:

- Black pepper is ground in water and the paste obtained is applied over the pimples. This produces local heat, redness and a burning sensation after which the pimple ruptures, the pus and infected blood within drains out and it heals without leaving behind a scar.

- Mustard seeds, acorus, lodh tree bark and rock salt are taken in equal quantities and powdered. This powder is mixed with requisite amount of water to make a paste which is applied to the face, to get rid of pimples.

- Silk cotton tree has thorns all over its body that resemble pimples in their physical appearance. The thorns of this tree are dried (dried thorns are readily available in the local Pansari shop) and ground in water to make a paste. This paste is applied to the pimples to obtain an early relief.

- The skin of an orange is crushed and ground well with added water and the pulp thus obtained is applied to the face. After a little while, the face is washed with lukewarm water.

- In olden days, it was a common practice of women to apply turmeric paste to the face before taking bath. This procedure leaves a yellow colour on the skin that makes it unpopular among the recent generation. Now, there is a solution for this.

Round zedoary is powdered and mixed with three times its quantity of channa powder or green gram flour.

The resulting powder is mixed with water and applied as a face pack. This medicine is very effective against pimples.

All the home remedies mentioned above are only applied locally. In addition, there are some medicines that can be consumed orally.

• Indian sarasaparilla is dried in sunlight and powdered. Half a spoon of powder is consumed two to three times a day along with lukewarm water. This brings about a cooling effect on the whole body and purifies the blood.

• Catechu is powdered and a quarter spoon of powder mixed with pure honey is consumed three times a day.

The following steps can be followed to prevent the recurrence of pimples.

• The face is kept clean and dry (oil free) by washing it three or four times a day with soap and warm water.

• When pimples appear, they should not be pricked with nails.

• Raw cucumber is consumed along with the skin as a whole daily during meals. This helps in purification of blood.

• Fried food and sweets are prohibited and consumed rarely.

• Physical exercises that bring about excessive sweating should be done everyday.

A balanced diet and a regular exercise regimen result in a glowing radiant skin.

LACK OF TASTE MAKES LIFE A WASTE

There are many people on this earth who "live to eat" rather than "eat to live". Their evergreen taste buds demand something new, everyday, all day long. The nose, salivary glands and tongue always work in unison. The smell of good food is just enough to set the saliva flowing and lips smacking. However, there are the unfortunate few who cannot even taste food with a good smell. These patients suffer from "dysguesia" or lack of taste which makes them feel that life is a waste.

There are many causes for this condition as described below:

• Excessive consumption of irritant beverages like coffee, tea, alcohol and cocoa cause acidity in the stomach and indigestion. This leads to abdominal discomfort, belching and difficulty in digesting food. As the condition progresses, the patient loses perception of taste. This condition is termed as dysguesia of gastritis.

• Excessive consumption of spicy food and fried food increases the acidity in the stomach causing heart burn, belching and abdominal discomfort. The belching is associated with a sense of sour and bitter taste in the mouth and ultimately loss of taste.

• Sneezing, running nose, blocked nasal passages, headache and other symptoms of common cold and respiratory infections present with a temporary loss of taste sensation. At times, the patient may also develop a sense of sweet or salt taste in the mouth leading to increased production of saliva and a sticky, frothy mouth.

MENTAL HEALTH

Though lack of taste may result from consumption of improper food and other co-existent diseases in the body, the state of mind of the patient is an extremely important cause. An imbalance in psychological health due to fear, anger, sorrow or depression also makes the food tasteless. Lack of taste may also be the side effect of certain medicines.

The home remedies for lack of taste are stated in Ayurveda as follows:

Ishtam Ishtaihi Saha Ashniyath

This means that "Food that is relished should be

eaten along with relatives and well-wishers". By adopting this golden line in daily life, many diseases of the digestive system and taste can be prevented forever.

Home remedies for lack of taste are stated in Ayurveda as follows:

• A quarter spoon each of cumin seeds and dry ginger are powdered and added to a vessel holding one cup of water. The solution is boiled and finally decanted. When warm, a pinch of common salt is added to it and the whole mouth is filled with the solution without swallowing. The chin is lifted and the solution is held in the mouth for two minutes and then spat out. This clears the mouth off slime and sticky saliva and stimulates the taste buds and the salivary glands.

• Dry gooseberry is powdered, added to a vessel holding two cups of water, boiled, cooled and decanted. The resulting solution is used as a mouth wash two to three times a day.

• The following home remedy is effective in loss of taste caused by gas and indigestion.

One elaichi and half a spoon of dry ginger powder are added to a vessel holding a cup of water and boiled. After thorough boiling, the solution is cooled and decanted. A pinch of asafoetida is added to the solution and consumed three times a day.

• Half a morsel of *pudina* leaves are washed in running water and crushed well. The crushed leaves are added to a vessel holding one cup of water and boiled. After decantation, the solution is held in the mouth for a while and then swallowed. This restores taste sensation and gives a pleasant smell to the breath.

• A quarter spoon of saunf seeds are well chewed and swallowed, three times a day.

• One spoon of dry gooseberry powder is consumed three times a day to restore taste sensation in cases of loss of taste due to stomach acidity. Similarly, glycyrrhiza powder consumed as described above restores taste sensation in cases of loss of taste due to excess body heat.

• In cases of taste loss due to common cold and respiratory infections, omum seeds powder mixed with pure honey is consumed three times a day.

In addition, dry ginger, pepper and long pepper are taken in equal quantities, powdered well and a quarter spoon of this powder mixed with honey is consumed three times a day.

• Dry ginger is cut into small pieces which are soaked in a vessel holding lime juice extract that is just enough to dip them in. A little salt is added to this and left overnight. The next day, the soaked ginger pieces are dried in sunlight. These medicated ginger pieces are called *Bhavana Shunti*. Three to four pieces of *Bhavana Shunti* are well chewed and swallowed three times a day to restore taste sensation and to improve appetite.

• Professional psychiatric counselling is a must for loss of taste due to mental ill health. Peace of mind, sympathy and consolation are the only medicines.

In addition, Indian pennywort leaves are washed well in running water, crushed and their juice is extracted. One spoon of juice mixed with a quarter cup of hot milk is consumed three times a day.

LOSS OF TASTE IN EXTREMES OF AGE

Infants, young children and elderly people constitute a sizeable number of patients suffering from the loss of taste.

Children with loss of taste are given to insufficient consumption of food. The following steps are essential for children as well as adults:

• Thorough and proper brushing of teeth twice daily.

• Compulsory mouth wash soon after eating chocolates, ice creams and sweets.

• Avoidance of irritant and very hot beverages.

It is interesting to note that children with worm infestation are also affected by loss of taste.

Dry embelia fruit is powdered and half a spoon of this powder mixed with honey is fed to the child before he goes to bed. This medicine restores taste sensation, improves appetite and kills worms.

Elderly people are advised to practise physical exercises suitable for their age and sex and to consume the right kind of food in the right quantity at right intervals of time.

The following home remedy holds promise for the elderly:

• Withania roots is cooked in milk and allowed to dry later. After complete drying, it is powdered and half a spoon of this powder is consumed with hot water three times a day. This medicine not only restores taste in the elderly, but also improves their appetite and strengthens their nervous system. Thus it almost gives them a new lease of life.

13

The Burning Stomach

Man is an integral part of nature. Hence, depending on seasonal variations, he consumes fruits and vegetables available in the season to protect his own health. When these seasonal foods are consumed in right quantities at right int[illegible]vals of time, there is no scope for any disease at all. Hence it is rightly said, "He who knows the right diet, knows no disease".

It is not wrong to say that the mouth is the gateway for a majority of diseases. Hence, any deviation from a healthy diet invariably leads to ill-health especially of the digestive system. The most common among such diseases is a burning sensation in the stomach referred to as stomach "hyperacidity". As this condition results from increase in *pittha* (body heat), it is called *Amlapittha* in Ayurveda. Excessive consumption of spicy and sour foodstuff increases the acid secretion in the stomach causing hyperacidity. As stated earlier, psychological ill health due to anxiety, fear, sorrow, tension etc., also cause stomach hyperacidity.

This condition is characterised by excessive belching with an unpleasant sour or bitter taste in the mouth, heartburn with a burning sensation in the centre of the chest, irritation and burning sensation in the throat and indigestion accompanied by abdominal discomfort, lethargy and weakness.

USHA PAANA: DRINK AT DAWN

Ayurveda says that consumption of half a stomachful of water corresponding to age and profession (Sedantary or manual labour) cures hyperacidity for life. *Usha* means "Dawn" and *Paana* means, "drink" and hence '*Usha paana*' means "Drink at dawn". This was a healthy practice adopted by our ancestors, of drinking two to three big cups of water early in the morning on an empty stomach which neutralised excess acidity in the stomach and relieved constipation.

The home remedies useful for hyperacidity are:
• Two spoons of sugar are dissolved in one cup of warm milk. Three seeds of black pepper are fried in pure ghee, powdered and added to the cup. After thorough stirring, the milk is consumed once a day. Frying in ghee reduces the spicy taste of black pepper and improves its digestive powers. Addition of sugar to milk decreases the acidity in the stomach.

• One morsel of green gram is mixed with water and a porridge is prepared. Two spoons of rice-corn powder and a little sugar are added to the porridge and mixed well. Consumption of this medicine three times a day, relieves stomach upset, abdominal discomfort, nausea, belching, dizziness and other symptoms of stomach hyperacidity.

• Five black raisins are soaked overnight in cold water. The grapes are squeezed and consumed early next morning on an empty stomach to get relief from hyperacidity. This home made medicine is also high on nutritive value and provides energy.

• Citrus fruit is cut and squeezed to extract the juice. To this is added half the quantity of *pudina* juice obtained by crushing its leaves. Finally, raw ginger juice is added to the above mixture of juices, in a quantity equal to half that of the *pudina* juice. An equal quantity of sugar is added and the whole mixture is heated over a low flame. With the evaporation of excess water, the mixture assumes a thicker consistency, after which it is poured into a glass bottle for storage. One spoon of this bottled medicine is dissolved in a quarter cup of cold water and consumed three times a day. This relieves the burning sensation in the throat, centre of the chest and the stomach. Citrus fruit is a concrete mixture of sour and bitter tastes and hence has powers of reducing stomach acidity. It is also used by pregnant women to relieve nausea and vomiting. Pudina leaves improve digestion and relieve abdominal discomfort. Although ginger has a bitter taste, when consumed in small quantities, it helps in digestion of the ingested food.

• One spoon of roasted and powdered coriander seeds are soaked overnight in a cup of cold water. The next morning, the water is decanted and consumed on an empty stomach to get relief from abdominal discomfort and dizziness. This home remedy is popularly known as *Dhanyaka Hima* and is very beneficial in all disorders caused by imbalance in *Pittha* or body heat.

Long term consumption of food stuff that cause imbalance in body heat (*Pittha*) increase hyper-acidity in the stomach, beyond tolerable limits, leading to the erosion of the protective covering on the inner layer of the stomach. This leads to irritation of the stomach, a condition called "Gastritis". This condition is characterised by the same symptoms as that of stomach hyperacidity. In addition it is associated with a sickening dis-comfort and hunger pangs in the region of the stomach when the stomach is empty.

The home remedies that combat gastritis are:

• Ash gourd is grated and squeezed to extract the juice. Consumption of half a cup of this juice three times a day, relieves stomach irritation as it reduces body heat.

• Glycyrrhiza root is powdered and one spoon of powder is mixed with half a cup each of milk and water. The whole mixture is brought to boil over a low flame till all the water content in it evaporates. It is then cooled, decanted and con-sumed three times a day. This reduces irritation in the stomach and prevents ulcer formation.

• A piece of bark of the red sandal tree is ground in water and half a spoon of the paste thus obtained is dissolved in half a cup of milk and consumed early in the morning on an empty stomach. This produces beneficial effects.

Though hyperacidity manifests itself with mild and general symptoms in the initial stages, if left untreated it produces stomach irritation, erosion and ulcer formation.

It is well known that there are six fundamental tastes viz. sweet, salt, sour, hard, hot (spicy) and bitter. According to Ayurveda, any food that has an excess of any of the above tastes should not be consumed. In particular, the foods rich in hot (spicy), sour and *masala* content should be consumed sparingly and in limited quantities, to prevent the disorders of the stomach.

MOTION SICKNESS

The smell of petrol or diesel, a bumpy ride on the road, air travel, road travel in hilly, mountainous areas bring about nausea and vomiting in few people. These people are said to be suffering from motion sickness.

A very light snack or meal before travel solves the problem. Hence travellers are advised not to travel either on an empty stomach or on a full stomach.

The following home remedies provide relief

• Elaichi seeds are chewed and the juice is swallowed frequently to stop motion sickness.

• Two spoons of *Madhiphala Rasayana*, a popular Ayurvedic medicine, can be consumed along with a quarter cup of cold water, just half an hour before the journey. It should be noted that *Madhiphala* is the synonymn of citrus fruit.

• Citrus fruit is cut and squeezed to obtain the juice. Equal amount of sugar and a little cumin seeds are added to the juice. The whole mixture is boiled till all the excess water content evaporates leaving behind a thick fluid. This is cooled and stored for future use in a glass bottle. One spoon of this medicine dissolved in a quarter cup of cold water is consumed three times a day to get relief from nausea and vomiting.

14

Jaundice – the yellow disease

In common parlance, there is a saying that goes – "A jaundiced eye sees the whole world yellow" referring to certain narrow-minded people with dated ideas, uncomfortable with changes in life. This apart, jaundice is actually defined as a symptom complex characterised by a yellow discolouration of the eye, skin and the body tissues. It is important to note that jaundice by itself is not a disease but only a symptom of an underlying disease in the body. The yellow colour is due to a substance that appears in the blood called bilirubin. This substance is a byproduct of the breakdown of the red blood corpuscles which form a very important and integral cellular component of the human blood. Jaundice is termed as *Kaamaala* in Ayurveda. This is a compound word with two components viz. *Kaama* and *la*.

Kaama refers to desire i.e., what the organs of special senses viz. eyes, nose, ears, tongue and skin desire to experience. *La* means no.

In totality *Kaamaala* refers to a condition in which the organs of special senses, especially, the tongue do not desire to taste even the choicest of foods. Though there are several causes of jaundice, those foods that cause imbalance in *Pittha* (body heat) are the most important.

In Ayurveda the different types of jaundice, attributed to various causes, have been classified under two main headings viz.

1. *Shakhashritha*

2. *Koshtashritha*

Home made medicines (Country medicine) have been extremely popular among jaundice patients. These medicines are of the following types:

1. Juice extracts of green leafy vegetables, consumed on an empty stomach.

2. Medicines that are applied into the eyes directly.

3. Needle therapy accompanied by chanting of hymns.

Exercise Caution!

According to modern medicine, jaundice can be broadly classified into two simple types

- A defect in the structure and/or the composition of the red blood corpuscles (described above) causes their premature destruction (normal life span of 120 days), raising the level of bilirubin in the blood and precipitating jaundice.

• Liver secretes a digestive juice called bile which facilitates the digestion of the fat content in food. Liver detoxifies the toxic bilirubin and releases it into the bile.

The bile flows from the liver into a pouch called gall bladder and from there through a narrow 'pipe' called 'common bile duct' into the intestines where it exerts its actions. Any obstruction in the flow of bile along this bile duct due to stone, cancerous growth, infection etc., raises bilirubin level in blood leading to jaundice.

In addition, infection of the liver called Hepatitis and hardening of liver called Cirrhosis also cause jaundice.

Elementary knowledge of the above two conditions is very helpful.

• Hepatitis—Five types are very well known viz. Hepatitis A, B, C, D and E of which types A and B deserve mention.

Hepatitis A is a food–borne infection caused by the consumption of food and water contaminated with Hepatitis A viruses. Hence, boiled and cooled water and hygienic preparation of food are the preventive measures.

• Hepatitis B is caused by blood transfusions, blood products like injectable serum, antibodies etc., unsafe sex, vaccines and injections, and accidental pricks from infected, unsterilised needles. Hence, doctors, hospital staff, lab personnel—any human being on earth is at equal risk of infection. Tests of blood and blood products, sterilisation, personal protection by using gloves, aprons etc., and safe sex are important preventive measures.

The common symptoms in a patient with jaundice in addition to yellow colour of the eye are the following:

a. Fever in case of hepatitis.

b. Lack of taste.

c. Lack of appetite.

d. Lethargy and weakness.

e. Dark yellow colour of urine and stools.

f. Pain in the right side of upper abdomen occasionally.

g. In advanced cases, yellow colour of tongue, mouth, skin and nails well made out in fair individuals.

h. In specific types, especially cirrhosis, there are bleeding disorders, blood vomiting and blood in the stools.

- Cirrhosis:

A condition in which the normal soft liver

becomes small and hard like a stone with the main culprit being uncontrolled alcoholism. Untreated Hepatitis B can also cause cirrhosis. It is a terminal disease. Patients have all symptoms of jaundice, bleeding disorders, blood vomiting, blood in stools, complete emaciation, distention of abdomen called "ascites" caused by obstruction of the blood flow in an important blood vessel, loss of hair, loss of sexual function, itching of skin, growth of breasts in men called "gynaecomastia", visible blood-vessels in the skin of the upper part of the body, all terminating in death.

A patient with cirrhosis is a living wreck.

Jaundice can be controlled by observing the following stringent measures:
1. Bedrest

2. A strict no-no to fried and oily food.

3. Consumption of large amounts of water.
Although country medicine is effective in the treatment of jaundice, it is not suitable for all types. Hence, jaundice patients should always consult a qualified doctor and turn to country medicine only after ascertaining that the jaundice is mild and not a complicated one.

Sugarcane juice prepared under hygienic conditions provides essential energy to the patients in the form of 'glucose' and wards off weakness. Jaundice patients should only be given rice porridge, fruit juice, water boiled and cooled, fat free butter milk and a bland diet. A fluid diet is always preferable.

The effective home remedies for jaundice are:

• A plant, six inches tall, called Frateromus is commonly found growing along the roadside. Although it has been effectively used as cure for wheezing in Ayurveda, it is also popular as a wonderdrug against jaundice.

Frateromus plant is uprooted (leaves, stem and root together), washed in running water, crushed and the juice extracted. Four spoons of this juice are mixed with one powdered elaichi and quarter spoon of cumin seed powder and the whole mixture along with a quarter cup of milk is consumed early in the morning on an empty stomach. This relieves the itching and improves appetite. Ultimately, the condition comes under control.

• The leaves of the tinospora creeper closely resemble that of the hugely popular decorative plant, the money plant. A three inch long stem of this creeper is crushed to extract the juice. The juice is mixed with equal quantity of honey and consumed three times a day. Immediately, jaundice comes under control and the fever, lethargy, weakness and loss of appetite are cured.

• The root of picrorrhiza is dried and powdered well. One spoon of powder mixed with honey is consumed early in the morning on an empty stomach. This medicine relieves constipation and helps in the outflow of accumulated bile-juice from the gall-bladder. This is the medicine of choice in gall-bladder diseases.

• Neem leaves are not only popular in controlling communicable diseases, but are also very effective in cases of jaundice. A bunch of neem leaves is washed in running water and crushed. Half a spoon of crushed leaves mixed with equal amount of honey is consumed three times a day. This medicine is especially effective against itching.

• There is misconception among people that turmeric, which is yellow in colour, should not be used in jaundice. This is truly baseless. As a matter of fact, turmeric is a very good medicine for jaundice. A thicker variety of turmeric called Indian Barberry is readily available. This is ground in water and a paste is obtained. A quarter spoon of the paste is consumed three times a day. This is extremely effective in controlling jaundice in children.

• Chebulic myloboron, beleric myloboron and dry gooseberry are all taken in equal quantities, their seeds are extracted and their outer shell (skin) is powdered. This powder is popularly known as *triphala churna*. One spoon of powder mixed with equal quantity of honey is consumed three times a day and effectively relieves fever, itching and constipation.

• *Bhringaraja* or Eclipta is a plant bearing white flowers and is a popular medication for hair growth. A handful of leaves of this plant are washed in running water, crushed and the juice is extracted. One spoon of the juice is consumed three times a day to ward off weakness and control jaundice effectively.

• Aloe is a plant that is commonly grown in the backyard and in gardens. The leaves of this plant have thick bear thorns along their margins and exude a thick gum-like "resin" when plucked. A few leaves are washed in running water and crushed to extract the juice. Two spoons of this juice are consumed three times a day. This medicine controls jaundice and is extremely effective in a majority of disorders of the gall-bladder.

• A rapidly growing plant called Spreading Hog Weed is commonly recognised as a part of stray vegetation. The raw root of the uprooted plant is cut, washed in running water and crushed to extract the juice. One spoon of this juice is consumed three times a day. The dried root of this plant, which is readily available, is powdered and one spoon of the powder is dissolved in one cup of milk and consumed three times a day. Since the patient recovers very soon from jaundice after taking this medicine, the plant is also called *Punarnava*. This is a compound word made up of *Punah* meaning again and *Nava* meaning new. This means, the patient is fit and fine again or he is rejuvenated.

• The leaves of dead nettle white plant are crushed and the juice thus extracted is decanted well. One drop of this juice is put into each eye of the jaundice patient. It is believed that this medicine increases tear production and helps in the fading of the yellow colour in the eye. Likewise, the juice extract of the leaves of several other plants are instilled in the eyes by the practitioners of village medicine or country medicine. But the eyes are very delicate organs and hence it is better to avoid using these unknown medicines.

It is very important to note that the yellow colour in the eye gradually fades away by itself within a few weeks after the cure of jaundice. Hence, no medicine needs to be put in the eye.

To conclude, bedrest and diet-control are an integral part of jaundice treatment and the supervision of a qualified doctor is a must.

15

Constipation and Piles—Born Together!

The word "constipation" sounds nightmarish to many. It is a product of an unhealthy lifestyle and is capable of assuming alarming proportions.

A little knowledge of the normal process of digestion makes understanding constipation easier. The food consumed is ground and churned in the stomach, after which the useful nutrients are absorbed into the blood in the small intestines and finally the unwanted component is converted into faeces (stools) and stored in the large intestine. As the large intestines fill, the stool is expelled at regular intervals by defecation. Imbalance in this normal process due to any reason results in constipation. Untreated constipation leads to many types of debilitating diseases.

Very often, constipation affects the elderly who complain of abdominal discomfort, bloating up of the stomach, heaviness of the whole body, lethargy, vomiting sensation, stomach ache and the like.

The main causes of constipation are:

- Inadequate consumption of water in a day. (Normal daily consumption should be at least 4-5 litres in an adult weighing 60 kgs.)

- Lack of regular physical exercise.

- Resisting the urge to defecate.

The only known important function of the large intestine is the absorption of water from the unwanted food materials that enter. Resisting the urge to defecate causes the stools to stay in the large intestine for a long time leading to absorption of nearly all its water content. This makes the stool hard, making it difficult and painful to pass. Water consumed in adequate quantity cures the problem.

Ayurveda states that buttermilk, milk and water, consumed in that order, cures constipation. Also, a cup of well-churned buttermilk is a must after meals because it helps in easy digestion of food. A cup of hot milk before going to bed induces sound sleep and helps in the easy passage of stool the next morning, preventing constipation. Consumption of a large amount of water, early in the morning on an empty stomach, increases the amount of water in the large intestines facilitating easy passage of stools.

Green leafy vegetables contain fibres and cellulose which are not digested by the human digestive system. Hence, the plant fibre and cellulose pass through all the parts of the digestive system untouched and constitute what is known as 'roughage' in the large intestines. The roughage mobilises the bowel (i.e. intestines) and helps in effortless passage of stools. Similarly, the seeds of fruits and vegetables consumed are undigested and add to the roughage, performing the above function. Hence, tomato, guava, brinjal, pomegranate, dry fig, grapes etc. which are full of seeds, should be frequently consumed. Warm water with a tender dry fig squeezed into it is taken to relieve constipation. In fact, papaya also induces bowel-movements. So also is banana which is available throughout the year.

The home remedies useful in cases of constipation are:

• There is a misconception among many that potato causes gas-formation and subsequently the muscles 'catch'. But, in fact it is a good bowel mobiliser. Constipation due to chronic, debilitating diseases is relieved by the consumption of one whole cooked potato along with the skin. This facilitates passage of stools and as a rich source of carbohydrates, it provides the much needed nutrition.

• One lime is cut and squeezed to extract the juice. The entire quantity of juice along with half a spoon of common salt is dissolved in two large cups of lukewarm water and consumed early in the morning on an empty stomach. This medicine instantly relieves constipation. In addition to stepping up digestion, the lime juice extract liquifies the hardened stools in the large intestine and facilitates its easy passage.

• The dried leaves of senna are powdered and mixed with equal quantity of powdered chebulic myloboron prepared after elimination of its seed. Half the above quantity of ("Sompu") Saunf and common salt are added and mixed well. One spoon of this mixture is dissolved in one cup of warm water and consumed at night.

• One spoon of Isabghol-husk powder should be dissolved in a cup of water and consumed at night. Another cup of water should be consumed soon after. "Isabghol-husk" is "hygroscopic" i.e., it has the property of absorbing water. Hence, on entering the large intestine, the "Isabghol-husk" absorbs water and swells, thereby expanding the large intestine and stimulating the urge to defecate. This also forms roughage and helps in easy passage of stools.

• Chebulic myloboron, beleric myloboron and dry gooseberry are taken in equal quantities, their seeds separated and their outer shells (skin) are powdered together. One spoon of the powder mixture is consumed with warm water before going to bed. This medicine not only relieves constipation but also stimulates the gall bladder.

• The use of castor oil to relieve constipation has been popular since ages. It is used extensively by both adults and children. Impure castor oil is detrimental to life. Hence, the castor oil used should be properly purified.

Self-medication of tablets prepared from croton seeds, is on the rise and can be detrimental to the patient's health and life. These tablets should be consumed under strict medical supervision only.

The bottomline is that constipation is preventable by adopting the following practices:

- A balanced diet

- Consumption of plenty of water.

- Consumption of abundant green leafy vegetables.

- Regular physical exercise according to age and sex.

PILES OR HAEMORRHOIDS

The dreaded consequence of neglected constipation is piles. This disorder affects the anal region (anus). A person suffering from piles keeps tossing up and down in his chair and cannot maintain his sitting posture for long. A sensation of needles pricking the anal region (anus) makes the patient change his posture at the drop of a hat. The condition is termed as *Arsha* in Ayurveda.

The causes of piles are many. But the most important is neglected constipation. In cases of constipation, the stool is stored in the large intestine for longer than normal. Hence, almost all the water in it is absorbed leaving the stool hard and rough. When this hard and rough stool passes out of the large intestine during defecation, it has to pass through the anal-passage. In the process, it exerts tremendous pressure and friction upon the blood vessels and the muscles of the anus, causing some of the blood vessels near the anus opening to stretch and protrude to the exterior. At times, the pressure and friction causes the rupture of these protruding blood-vessels, leading to the passage of blood in stools.

Ayurveda states that the *Dharana* and *Udheerana* of the normal bowel-movements (urge to defecate) is responsible for piles. The resistance of the urge to defecate at any point of time due to unfavourable social circumstances and environment is given the name *Dharana*. Voluntary application of pressure over the lower abdomen and forceful expulsion of stool is given the name *Udheerana*. Both the habits are worth giving up.

Excessive consumption of spicy food, inadequate water intake and sedentary lifestyle predispose to the appearance of piles.

Piles are of two types viz.
a. *Bahya* meaning external and

b. *Abhyantara* meaning internal.
Ayurveda states that this condition is treated only in the following order of preference:
- Oral medicines (*Oushadha*).

• Application of irritants (*Kshara*).

• Cauterization (*Agni*).

• Surgery (*Shasthra Chikitsa*).

In the initial stages of the disorder, piles is treated by medicines consumed orally and by those applied locally in and around the anus. At this stage, these medicines may be effective.

In piles that is undeterred by the above treatment, *Kshara* holds promise. In *Kshara* treatment, some herbs with caustic properties are burnt and their ashes are mixed with water to make a paste. The paste is smeared along the entire length of a clean thread. This pre-medicated thread is tied to the protruding blood vessels which dry up and wither away in course of time, curing the disorder.

In ancient times, a red-hot iron rod was used to burn the protruding blood-vessels. This was called *Agni Chikitsa*.

Finally, the surgical treatment for piles has been elaborated in the great book *Sushrutha Samhitha*, the surgical text of Ayurveda, written by Sushrutha Maharshi, the Father of Surgery.

The home remedies useful in piles are:

• Yam is cut into small pieces, dried and powdered. This medicine arrests bleeding and relieves constipation associated with piles. Ayurveda states that this vegetable should be consumed especially by piles patients both as a medicine and as regular food.

• The juice extracts of crushed alternanthera and crushed radish leaves are mixed in equal quantities and a pinch of rock salt is added to the mixture. This medicine should be taken twice daily.

• Two spoons of powdered dry gooseberry are dissolved in butter milk and consumed early in the morning on an empty stomach. This home remedy helps in arresting bleeding.

• The seed of chebulic myloboron is disposed off and its outer shell (skin) is powdered. Half a spoon of this powder is mixed with equal quantity of powdered old jaggery and consumed twice daily. This medicine relieves constipation, abdominal discomfort and indigestion.

• Touch-me-not plant is uprooted as a whole (leaves, stem and roots together), washed in running water and crushed to extract the juice. One spoon of this juice is mixed with a little amount of boiled and cooled milk and consumed twice daily. As stated elsewhere, touch-me-not plant has styptic (stop-bleeding) properties that help in arresting bleeding and in controlling piles.

• Turmeric is ground in water and its paste is mixed with a little rock salt and applied to the protruding blood vessel at the anus. Turmeric has antiseptic properties that bring down the swelling in the region of the anus and prevents any possible infection.

• Drumstick leaves and radish leaves are taken in equal proportions and ground together thoroughly. After slight warming over a low flame, the ground leaves are applied to the protruding blood vessels at the anus. This provides instant relief from pain.

• Powdered turmeric is mixed with a little castor-oil and the paste thus obtained is warmed over a low flame and applied to the protruding blood vessels at the anus. This reduces the pain and swelling in the region of piles.

The following are the preventive measures against occurrence/recurrence of piles:

a. Consumption of well churned buttermilk.

b. Strict adherence to a healthy diet and adequate water consumption to prevent constipation.

c. Dipping the anus in a tub of warm water for half an hour three times a day.

When the above medicines fail to provide relief the consultation of a qualified doctor is necessary.

To conclude, I wish to tell my esteemed readers that–If face is the index of the mind, then digestive system is the index of our health. The tongue heads the list of wanted culprits and the mouth is the door broken in by diseases.

Hence, to lead a healthy life, my dear readers, eat to live but do not live to eat!

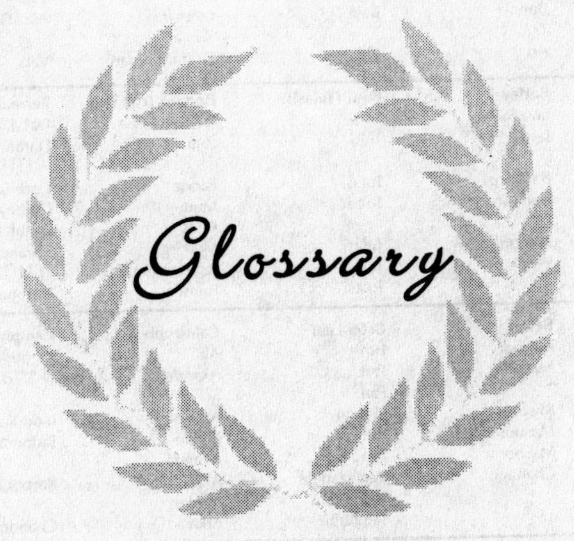

Glossary

	Acasia	Acorus	Aloe	Banyan Tree
Hindi	Biswul	Bach	Ghikanvar	Bor
Bengali	Kuchui	Bach	Grita Kumari	Bar
Punjabi				Bor
Tamil	Indu	Vashambu	Chirukattali, Kattalai	Pudavam
Telugu	Karusikaya	Vadaja	Chinna-Kata Banda	Peddamatti
Marathi		Vaj		Vad/Vada
Kannada	Banni	Baje	Lolesara	Ala
Malayalam			Kumari	
Sanskrit	Ari	Bhadra	Gritha-Kumari	Vata

	Barley	Basil (Tulasi)	Bastard Teak Tree	Bermuda Grass
Hindi	Java/Jo/Jou	Tulsi	Dhak/Palas	Dab/Durva
Bengali	Java	Tulsi	Palas	Darbha/Kusha
Punjabi				
Tamil	Bali-Arisi	Tulasi	Parasa	Darbha
Telugu	Yava-dhanya	Tulasi	Moduga	Darbha
Marathi	Java		Palas	Darbha
Kannada	Javegodhi	Tulasi	Muthuga	Garake-hullu
Malayalam		Tulasi	Palasinsa-matha	
Sanskrit		Tulasi	Palasha	Darbha/Kusha

	Besan	Betel Leaf	Calotropis	Camphor
Hindi	Masoor	Pan	Ak	Karpur
Bengali	Masoori	Pan	Akanda	
Punjabi		Pan		
Tamil	Misoor	Vettilai	Arkkam	Indu/Karppuram
Telugu	Masoor-Pappu	Vitika	Jilledu	Karpuramu
Marathi	Masoor	Pan	Akanda	
Kannada	Chanagi	Veelyaadele	Akka	Karpura
Malayalam		Tambulam	Arikku	
Sanskrit		Tambulli	Arka	Chandraha

	Catechu	Celosia	Clove	Common/Crystal Salt
Hindi	Arvi	Sufaid-murgha	Laung	Panganamak
Bengali	Kachu	Swet-murga	Lavanga	
Punjabi		Sarwali	Laung	
Tamil	Seppan-Kizhangu/ Shamakkilangu		Krambu	Uppu
Telugu	Chamadumpa	Gurugu		Uppu
Marathi	Kachualu	Kurdu	Lavang	
Kannada	Kachu	Anne	Lavanga	Samudralavana
Malayalam	Shembu			Dronilavanam
Sanskrit	Kachu	Vitunna	Lavanga	

	Cotton	Croton Seeds	Cumin Seeds	Dhatura
Hindi	Kapas	Jamalgota	Jira/Zira	Sadah-Dhatura
Bengali		Jaypal	Jira	Dhatura
Punjabi				Tattu-dattura
Tamil	Parutthi	Nervalam	Shiragam	Vellum-mattai/Umaitai
Telugu	Patthi	Nepala	Jiraka	
Marathi		Jamalgota		Dhutura
Kannada	Hatthi-gida	Japala	Jeerige	Ummathi
Malayalam		Nervalam	Jorekam	
Sanskrit	Pichuhu	Jayapala	Jiraka	Dhustura

	Dead Nettle White	Eclipta	Elaichi	Eucalyptus
Hindi	Chota-halkusa	Bhangra	Choti-elaichi	
Bengali	Chota-halkusa	Kesuti/Kesuria	Choti-elaichi	
Punjabi	Tattu-dhatura			
Tamil	Tumbai	Garuga	Yelakkai	Talanoppi
Telugu	Tummachettu	Galagara	Yelakkayalu	
Marathi	Tamba	Maka	Elachi	Nilgiri
Kannada	Tumbe	Bringaraja	Elakki	Karpura-maram
Malayalam				
Sanskrit	Dronapushpi	Bringaraja/Kesaraja	Ela	

	Frateromus/ Phyllanthus	Gingiley	Glycyrrhiza	Gooseberry
Hindi	Jar-amla	Til	Jathimadh/Mulhatti	Amla/Aonla
Bengali	Bhui-amla	Til	Jashti-madhu	Amla/Amlaki
Punjabi			Muleti	
Tamil	Kilkkaynelli	Yelluchedi	Atimaduram	Nelli
Telugu	Nelavusari	Nuvvulu	Athimaduramu	Amalakamu
Marathi	Bhui-avala	Til	Jashti-madhu	
Kannada	Nela-Nelli	Ellu	Atimadura/ Jyeshta-madhu	Amalaka/Nellikai
Malayalam	Kizhkkayinelli	Ellu		Nelli
Sanskrit	Bhumyamalaki	Tila	Yashti-madhu	Adiphala/Amalaka

	Henna	Honey	Indian Liquorice	Indian Pennywort
Hindi	Hena/Mehndi	Shahad	Ghuhchi/Rati	Brahmi
Bengali	Mehedi/Mendi		Kunch	Brihmi-sak
Punjabi	Mendi			
Tamil	Marudondri	Tihen	Gundumani	Nir-brahmi
Telugu	Gorinta	Then	Gariginja	Brahmi
Marathi	Mehndi		Gunja	
Kannada	Goranti	Jenu-thuppa	Gulaganji	Ondelaga/Brahmi
Malayalam	Mayilanji		Kakani	Nir-Brahmi
Sanskrit	Mendika	Makshika	Gunja	Nira-Brahmi

	Indian Sarasaparilla	Khulanjan	Lac	Liquorice
Hindi	Magrabu	Khulinjan	Lakh	Jathimadh/Mulhatti
Bengali	Anantamul	Sugandha-bacha		Jashti-Madhu
Punjabi				Muleti
Tamil	Nannari		Arakka	Atimaduram
Telugu	Gadhisugandhi		Lekka	Atimaduramu
Marathi	Anantamul/Uparsara			Jashti-madhu
Kannada	Sogade-beru	Rashme	Aragu	Atimadura/Jyeshtamadh
Malayalam	Nannari			
Sanskrit	Anantha	Yashti-Madhu	Vrikshamaya	

	Lodh Tree	Long Pepper	Malabar Tamarind	Mustard
Hindi	Lodh	Piplamul	Kokam	Kali Sarson
Bengali	Lodh	Piplamul		Kali sarson
Punjabi	Lodar	Piplamul		
Tamil			Murgal	Karuppu-kkadugu
Telugu	Lodduga	Pippalu		Nallaavalu
Marathi	Lodh	Piplamul	Beerund	
Kannada	Lodhra	Pippali	Murginahuli	Sasive
Malayalam				Karupakatuka
Sanskrit	Lodhra	Pippali		Kala-Sarshapa

	Nerium	Peepal Tree	Pepper	Picrorrhiza
Hindi	Kaner	Pipal	Gol Mirch	Katki/Kuru
Bengali	Karabhi	Asvattha	Gol Mirch	Katki/Kuru
Punjabi	Kaner	Pipal		Karru
Tamil	Karaviram	Arasu	Milagu	Katukuragani
Telugu	Karaviram	Pippali	Marichamu	Katukurogani
Marathi	Kanhera	Pipal	Kalamiri	Kalikutki
Kannada	Nanjabattalu	Arali	Menasu	Katukarohini
Malayalam	Karaviram		Kurumulaka	Katukhurohani
Sanskrit	Karavira	Pippala	Maricha	Katuka

	Plumbago	Red Sandal	Rock Salt	Round Zedoary
Hindi	Lal-chitra	Lal Chandan	Sendha Namak	Jangli Haldi
Bengali	Lal-chitra	Rakta Chandana		Ban-Halud
Punjabi	Chitrak			
Tamil	Akkini/Sittragam	Sensandanam	Saindavalavanam	Kasturi Manjal
Telugu	Errachitramulam	Raktachandanamu	Saindavalavanamu	Kasturi Manjal
Marathi	Lal-chitra	Raktachandan		Ran-hald
Kannada	Chitramula	Raktachandana	Saindavalavana	Kasturi-Arishina
Malayalam	Chettikotuveli	Raktachandanam	.	
Sanskrit	Chitraka	Raktachandana	Sindhuttam	Vanaharidar

	Sandal	Saunf	Senna	Silk Cotton Tree
Hindi	Chandan	Saonf	Hindisana	Simul
Bengali	Chandan	Muhuri	Sanna-makki	Rokto-Simul
Punjabi	Chandan			
Tamil	Ingam	Shombu	Nilavirai	Purani
Telugu	Chandanamu		Nela-tangedu	Salmali
Marathi	Chandan	Sonf	Sonamukhi	Semul
Kannada	Chandana	Sompu	Sonamukhi	Booruga
Malayalam	Chandanam		Nilavaka	Mocha
Sanskrit	Chandana	Shetapusapa	Sonamukhi	Salmili

	Spreading Hogweed	Sweet Flag	Sweet Gruel	Til/Gingiley
Hindi	Sant	Bach	Kheer	Til
Bengali	Punarnava	Bach		Til
Punjabi			Kheer	
Tamil	Mukaratte-kirei	Vashambu	Payasam	Yelluchedi
Telugu	Punaranva	Vadaja	Payasamu	Nuvvulu
Marathi	Ghetulli	Vaj		Til
Kannada	Komme	Baje	Payasa	Ellu
Malayalam			Payasam	Ellu
Sanskrit	Punarnava/ rakta-punarnava	Bhadra	Payasah	Tila

	Tinospora	Turmeric	Withania
Hindi	Giloe/Gulancha	Haldi	Akri
Bengali	Giloe/Gulancha	Haldi	Ashvagandha
Punjabi	Gilo		Khamgira
Tamil	Sintal	Manjal	Amukkura
Telugu	Somida	Pasupu	Pennerugadda
Marathi	Gulwel		Kaknaj
Kannada	Amrita-balli/Ondelaga	Arishina	Asvagandhi
Malayalam	Sittamrytu		
Sanskrit	Guduchi	Haridra	Ashwagandha

VEGETABLES

	Ash Gourd	Beans	Bitter Gourd	Drumstick
Hindi	Pela	Nishpara	Karela	Soanjna
Bengali	Haldi	Makhanasim	Karala	Saina
Punjabi			Karela	Soanjna
Tamil	Kalyana-poochuni	Mochai	Parakkachedi/Pagel	Murungai
Telugu	Gummadi	Anumul	Kakara	Sajana
Marathi		Pavate	Karla	Sujna
Kannada	Boodhugumbala	Avarekai	Hagalakai	Nugge
Malayalam			Kappakka	Sigru
Sanskrit	Valliphala		Sushavi	Sobhanjana

	Garlic	Ginger	Green Peas	Nutgrass Tubers
Hindi	Lasan/lasun	Adrak	Mattar	Motha/Mutha
Bengali	Lasan/lasun	Ada	Matar	Motha/Mutha
Punjabi		Adrak		
Tamil	Vellaipundu	Inji	Patani	Korai
Telugu	Velluli	Adrakamu	Gundusanagalu	Tungamuste
Marathi	Lasan/lasun	Adu	Vatane	Musta
Kannada	Belluli	Shunti	Batani	Konnarigedde
Malayalam	Velluli	Andrakam		
Sanskrit	Lashuna	Ardraka		Musta

	Onion	Radish	Snake Gourd	Yam
Hindi	Piyaz	Muli	Chachinga	Amaltas
Bengali	Piyaj	Mula	Chichinga	Sundali
Punjabi		Muli	Chichinda	
Tamil	Irulli/Vengayam	Mullangi	Pudel	Konnei
Telugu	Nirulli	Mullangi	Lingapotla	Rela
Marathi	Kanada	Mula	Pandolu	Bhava
Kannada	Irulli	Mulangi	Padavala	Suvarnagedde
Malayalam		Mullangi		
Sanskrit	Palandu	Mulaka	Chichinda	Suvarnaka

GREEN LEAFY VEGETABLES

	Adhatoda/Vasaka	Alternanthera	Asparagus	Basella
Hindi	Adulasa		Satawar	Lalbachlu/poi
Bengali	Bakas	Kanchari	Shatamuli	Rakto-pui/Poi
Punjabi				
Tamil	Adadodai	Ponnaganni-Keeray	Shimai-shadavari	Pasalei/Vaslakkirai
Telugu	Adasasamu	Ponnaganta-Kura	Challa-gadda	Batsala
Marathi	Adulasa		Satavari	Velgond
Kannada	Adusoge	Honagonesoppu	Shatavari	Basale
Malayalam		Ponnanganni-keeray	Shatavali	Basala
Sanskrit	Vasaka		Shatamuli	Potaki/Putika

	Coriander	Mentha/Pudina	Ruta	Sesbania
Hindi	Dhanya/Dhania	Podina	Nagphana	Basna
Bengali	Dhane	Podina	Nagphana	Bak
Punjabi				
Tamil	Kothamalli	Pudina	Ngadali	Agatti
Telugu	Dhaniyalu	Pudina	Nagadali	Agise
Marathi		Pudinah	Samar	Basna
Kannada	Kotthamban	Pudina	Nagadali	Agase
Malayalam	Kothumpalari	Putiyina	Nagamulla	Akatti
Sanskrit	Dhanyaka	Pudinah	Vidara	Agasti

CEREALS

	Dil	Black Gram	Channa Dal	Green Gram
Hindi	Saunf	Urid	Chana	Mung-dal
Bengali		Mashkalai	Chola	Mung-dal
Punjabi		Mash	Chola	Mung-dal
Tamil	Shombu	Paunippayaru	Kadalai	Patchaipayaru
Telugu	Sompu	Patchapesalu	Sanagalu	Wuthulu
Marathi		Udid/Ulundu	Chana	Mung-dal
Kannada	Sabbasige (Sadap)	Uddu	Kadale	Hesaru-bele
Malayalam		Cherupoyara		
Sanskrit	Mishihi	Masha	Chanaka	Mudga

	Horse Gram	Jowar	Omum	Ragi
Hindi	Kulthi/Koolthee	Joar/Jowar	Ajowan	Mandua/Mandal
Bengali	Kurti-kalia	Joar/Jowar	Jowan	Marua
Punjabi		Joar/Jowar		
Tamil	Kollu	Cholam	Omum	Kelvaregu
Telugu	Ulavalu	Jonnalu	Omamu	Ragulu
Marathi	Kulthi/Koolthee	Joar/Jowar	Ajwan	Nagli
Kannada	Hurali	Jolah	Omu	Ragi
Malayalam	Muthiva	Chavela		
Sanskrit	Kulattha	Dirghamala	Ajamoda	Ragi/Rajika

	Red Toor Dal	Trigonella/Methi	Whole Black Gram
Hindi	Arahad/Toor	Methi	Urid
Bengali	Aairi/Adar	Methi	Mashkalai
Punjabi		Methi	Mash
Tamil	Thovaria	Vendayam	Ulundu/Paunippayaru
Telugu	Kandulu	Mentulu	Patchapesalu
Marathi	Thuri/Toor	Methi	Udid
Kannada	Thogari-bele	Menthya	Uddina-kalu
Malayalam		Ventayam	Cherupoyara
Sanskrit		Methi	Masha

NUTS

	Arecanut	Beleric-myloboron	Chebulic-myloboron	Coconut
Hindi	Supari	Bahera	Harir	Nariyal
Bengali	Supari	Bahera	Haritaki	Dab/Narikel
Punjabi		Bahera		
Tamil	Kamugu/Pakku	Akkam/Tandi	Kadukkai	Tenkai
Telugu	Vakka	Tandra	Karitaki	Narikelamu
Marathi	Sopari	Behara	Hirda	Narel
Kannada	Adike	Tarekai	Alalekai	Tengu
Malayalam	Adakka	Tusham	Katukku	Narikelam
Sanskrit	Poogiphalam	Bahira	Haritaki	Narikela

FRUITS

	Emblic-myloboron	Nutmeg	Country Fig	Dry Fig
Hindi	Baberang	Jaiphal	Gular	Anjiri/Anjir
Bengali	Biranga	Jaiphal	Jagya-dumur	Anjir
Punjabi	Babrung		Kumbal	Fagari
Tamil	Vayuvidanga	Jadikkay	Atti	Simaiyatti
Telugu	Vayuvidanga	Jajikaya	Atti	Anjuru/Medi
Marathi	Vaivarang/Vavadinga	Jaiphal	Umbar	Anira
Kannada	Vayuvidanga	Jayi-kayi	Atthi	Anjura
Malayalam		Jatikka	Atti	
Sanskrit	Vidanga	Jatiphala	Udumbara	Anjira

	Dry Grapes	Jamboo Fruit	Lime	Mango
Hindi	Angur	Jamun	Nimbu	Am/Amb
Bengali	Angur	Jam	Nimbu	Am
Punjabi	Angur			Am
Tamil	Trachei/Kottani	Neredam	Vepa	Mamaram
Telugu	Draksha	Jambuvu	Vepa	Amramu
Marathi	Drakh	Jambu	Nimbu	Am/Amb
Kannada	Drakshi	Nerale	Nimbe	Mavu
Malayalam	Gostani	Naval	Vepa	Amram
Sanskrit	Draksha	Jambu	Nimba	Amra

FLOWERS

	Pomegranate	White Fig	Jasmine	Marigold
Hindi	Anar-ke-per	Pilkhan	Motia/Mugra	
Bengali	Dalimgachh	Pakar	Bel/Mogra	
Punjabi	Anar	Pikhan		Zergul
Tamil	Madalai	Kurugu	Malligai	
Telugu	Dalimma	Badijuvvi	Bondumall	
Marathi	Dalimba	Pipli	Mogri	
Kannada	Dalimbe	Basari	Mallige	Chendu-hoovu
Malayalam	Dadiman	Pepar	Mulla	
Sanskrit	Dadima	Plaksha	Mallika